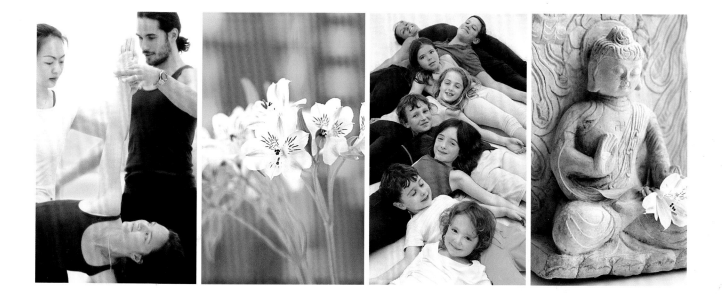

everyone try yoga

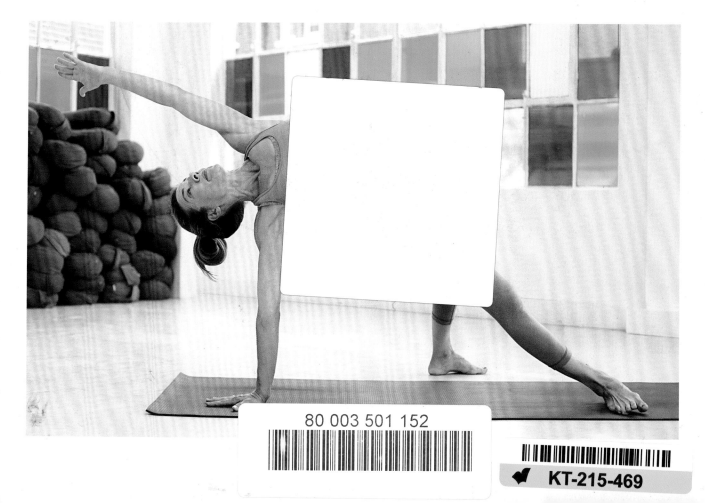

everyone try yoga

finding your yoga fit

by Victoria Woodhall
with Jonathan Sattin
and triyoga

photography by Clare Park

KYLE BOOKS

First published in Great Britain in 2013 by
Kyle Books
An imprint of Kyle Cathie Ltd
23 Howland Street, London W1T 4AY
general.enquiries@kylebooks.com
www.kylebooks.com

ISBN: 978-0-85783-071-5

Editor: Catharine Robertson
Designer: Angela Lamb
Photographer: Clare Park
Photographer's Assistant: Matthew Tugwell
Hair & Make-up: Marie Coulter
Copy Editor: Liz Murray
Proofreader: Ruth Baldwin
Production: Lisa Pinnell

* Except those credited on page 189.

A Cataloguing In Publication record for this title is available from the British Library.
Colour reproduction by Alta Image
Printed and bound in China by C&C Offset Printing Company Ltd.

DISCLAIMER: The authors and publisher cannot accept any responsibility for
misadventure resulting from the practice of any of the exercises in this book. It is
not intended and should not be used as guidance for the treatment of serious
health problems; please refer to a medical professional if you have concerns about
any aspect of your condition or fitness level.

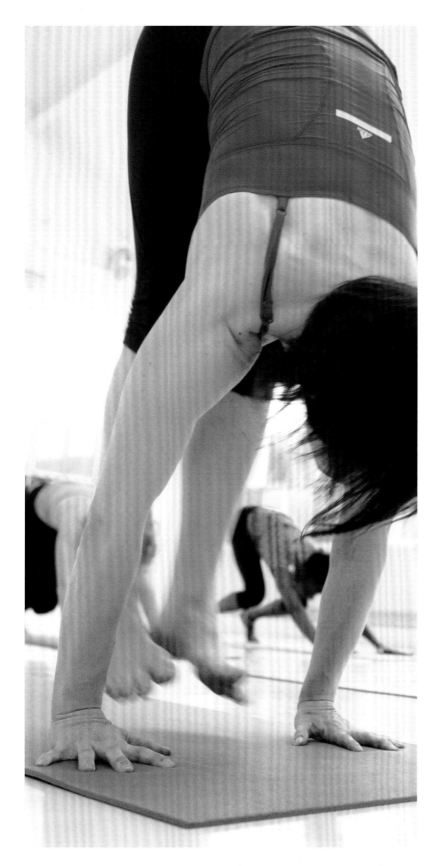

contents

the triyoga story

by Jonathan Sattin

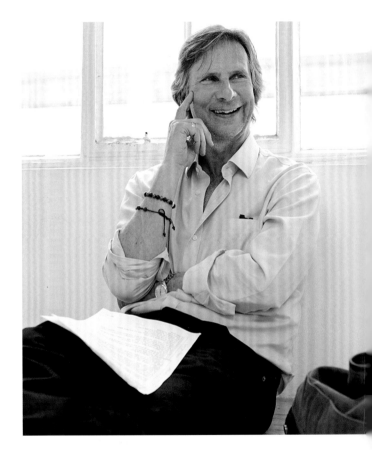

It was 1985 and I was a walking cliché – a senior partner in a West End law practice, smoking 40 Marlboro a day and drinking 14 mugs of coffee (with at least two sugars). Exercise consisted of playing competitive football and tennis and non-competitive walking my dog. I worried about my health and stress – counteracted by worrying some more and having jasmine tea with my morning cigarette. I'd tried yoga and meditation on and off and had even bought a book but got no further than the contents page. My football team-mates used to take the proverbial – and my end-of-season T-shirt had 'guru' written on it.

One of the partners in my law firm suggested I try a yoga class that his wife had been going to. I booked myself in for a one-on-one lesson; as I lay on the mat with my eyes closed, I could see a wall of mirrors and myself running away from it. I knew it was time to stop and take a look. Somehow I knew yoga was the key.

I started practising with a teacher called John Stirk (see page 86) once a week. And, without my noticing, my life began to change. I didn't suddenly give up being a lawyer (that came later) or shave my head. I still worried about my health and stress levels, but I was doing something about them. I could see that yoga was a pretty effective detox. There were times when I sweated so much in class that I could almost feel the nicotine coming through my skin. Within weeks I had given up cigarettes and coffee. I picked up my meditation practice. I was introduced to the meditation teacher Gurumayi and began to see that yoga had a much bigger reach than just the physical. I meditated

more regularly and started to trust my instincts as a lawyer as well as my knowledge. My football improved (or so I thought) and I was still very competitive, not just because of the physical shape I was in (full lotus position always throws opponents) but here too, my instincts felt sharpened.

In 1996 I came up with a concept of a holistic health club. I wanted to call it Tribeca because it sounded cool and very 'New York'. The project didn't come off, but

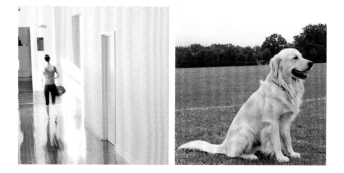

some friends said, 'Why not do what you love – yoga?' Tribeca became triyoga. Suddenly there was a different impetus. We wanted to create the highest-quality centre for true wellbeing, combining yoga, pilates and treatments. triyoga, in Primrose Hill, London opened on 19 February 2000. On that day we offered free classes to everyone, thinking that no one would come. But there was a queue from our mews into the street. Through a truly welcoming environment we wanted to dispel the illusion about who could practise yoga. You didn't need to be a supple, size six, 25-year-old female and eat tofu. It was for everyone, including the stressed-out, the desk-bound and those who played sports but paradoxically couldn't touch their toes. Yoga was for everyone. 'Everyone triyoga' became our slogan, because we meant it.

Our aim was to have the best teachers offering a broad range of authentic yoga styles, so that everyone could find a class that suited them. We wanted to honour the tradition of yoga – not just what we do on the mat, but how we live our lives. We wanted to provide a space where the many different styles of yoga could coexist, giving as many people as possible the chance to find an entry point to yoga and having fun on the way.

We invited the world's leading teachers to hold guest workshops. Ashtanga pioneer John Scott was the first. He continues to come back every year, to everyone's delight. We now welcome the top international teachers – Sarah Powers, Gurmukh, David Swenson, Max Strom and many more. Now in our second decade, we have four London centres and a thriving teacher-

training programme. In honour of my golden retriever and friend, Teddy (above), who was in charge of greeting from our opening until 2007, we launched the Teddy Foundation to help provide yoga for all children.

But thanks for our success goes most of all to our inspiring triyoga teachers, because of whom triyoga has consistently remained a centre of excellence. And it's thanks to them that this book has come together. They have given their time and wisdom in order to share the many practices of and approaches to yoga – to inspire you to begin or to progress your yoga journey.

Ironically for someone who owns a yoga business, my practice these days isn't as regular as I'd like. Sometimes I go to two classes a week. Sometimes I practise at home every day for 20 minutes, sometimes not for weeks. Even after 25 years, it's still a game between 'what's good for me' and 'what's stopping me'. But yoga is now the way I live my life. The key is just to keep showing up on the mat whenever I can.

A few years ago I was in reception at triyoga Primrose Hill and I saw one of my old football team-mates, who had been practising yoga with us for a few years. Of all the guys from our victorious 'championship' team we are the only two still playing and of course we still think (or dream) that we're really good.

So for this book, our intention is to give you a flavour of triyoga; so you can choose what would work best for you from a great range of styles, learn from the very best teachers and have fun on the way.

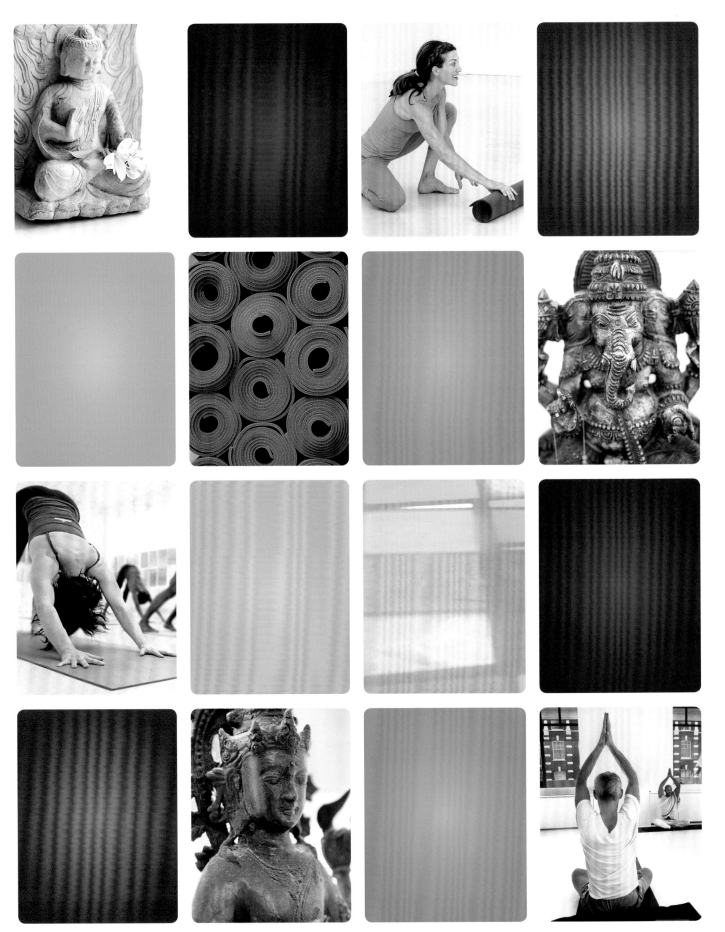

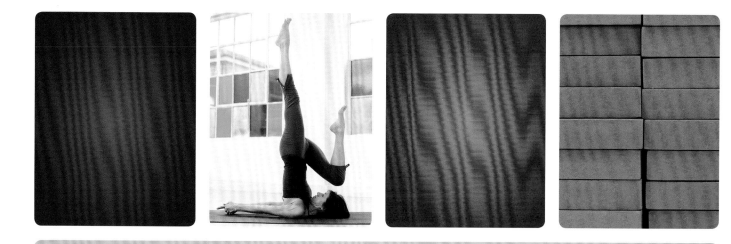

what is yoga?

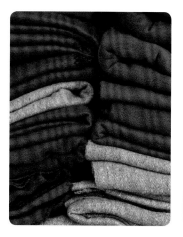
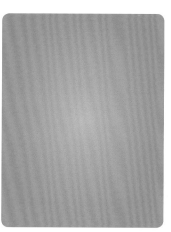
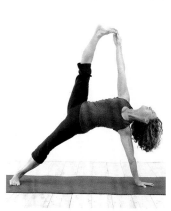

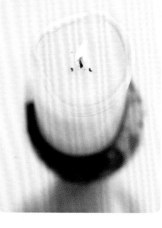
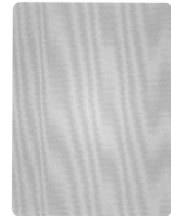
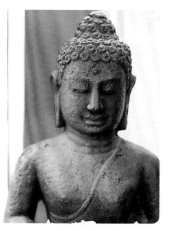

yoga: *the perfect antidote to the modern world*

What if you were told that there was a pill that could give you better sleep, more energy and enhance your powers of concentration? You'd probably stop what you were doing, and want to know more...

BY VICTORIA WOODHALL

Then what if you discovered that that pill could also tone your body, help you lose weight, make you look and feel younger, keep you limber in old age, boost your immune system and improve your running/tennis/football?

But that's not all. This pill can change how you feel. It can help you work out who you are and where you are going; it can help you feel happier in your own skin.

So where's the catch? There isn't one. In fact, anyone can take it regardless of age, race, gender or physical ability. What's more, there are absolutely no side-effects (unless you count possibly adding a couple of centimetres to your height, losing the taste for junk food and making a few new like-minded friends).

Sounds like a no-brainer. Of course you'd like one of these pills, please. In fact, you'd like a lifetime's supply for yourself and for your friends and family as well.

OK, so we weren't telling the complete truth. There is a catch. A couple of times a week, depending on how quickly you wanted all these wonderful benefits to start working, you would have to queue for about an hour to get the pill. Would you still do it? On balance, yes.

Now while you are waiting in line, you have to take your shoes off, get on a mat and do a bit of stretching, deep breathing and some lying down at the end. Then you get your pill. How hard can it be?

That's it. That's all you have to do. So are you in? Hmmm, not sure?

Here's the thing; most of us experience resistance to something that might be good for us, especially if it involves effort or change. Sometimes it's much easier to carry on as we are, to say we don't have time. That way we don't have to address what it is that's stopping us.

But there's no need to overthink it; just turn up and give it a try. Oh, and did we mention that it's also fun?

So now are you in? Great! Welcome to the new improved you.

By now you will have worked out that there is no such pill, of course, and if there were, it would have no more life-enhancing properties than a sugar lump. But the mat is very real. And what we rather flippantly referred to as 'a bit of stretching, deep breathing and lying down' is actually a very ancient discipline, one that can potentially bring you all the benefits of this fictitious pill. It's not an overnight miracle cure; it's a journey, but the effects can last a lifetime. It's yoga.

It's not an overnight miracle cure; it's a journey, but the effects can last a lifetime.

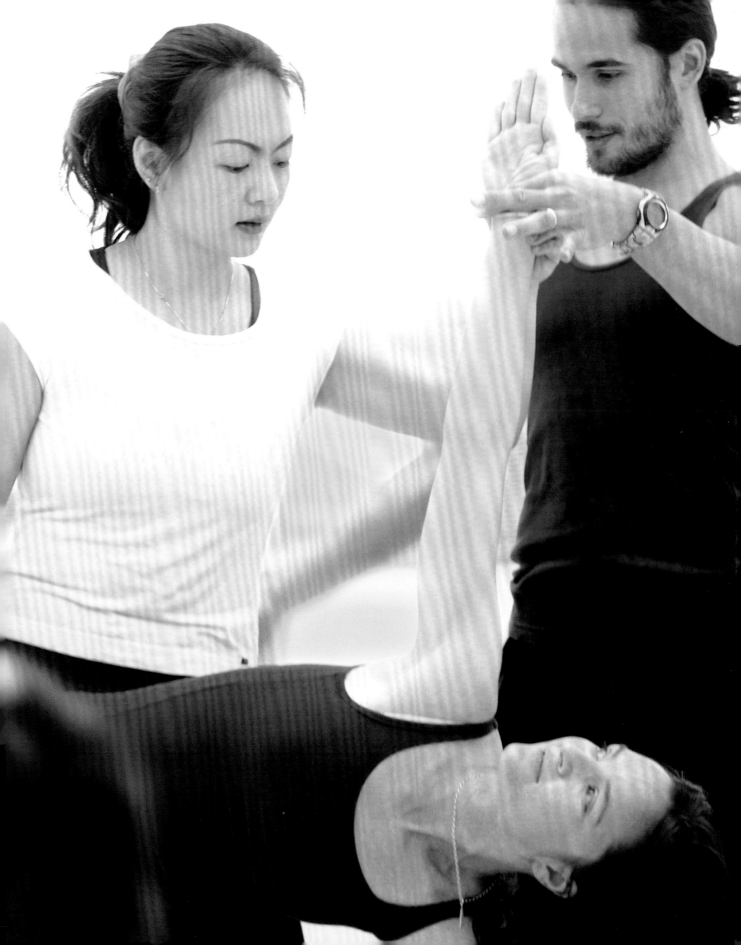

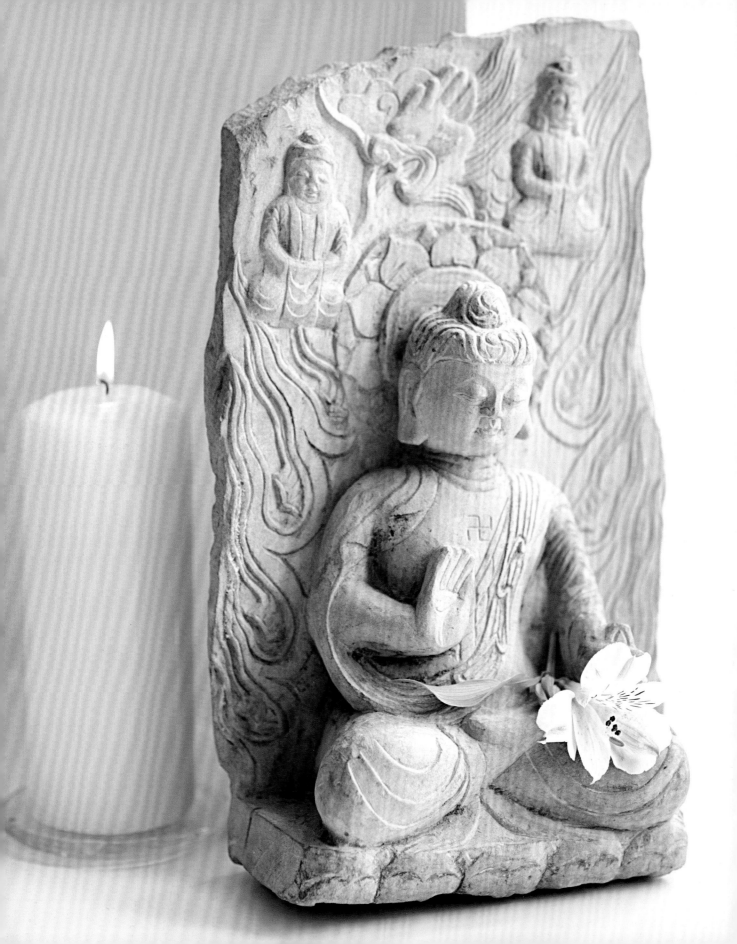

WHERE DOES YOGA COME FROM?

Yoga practice is so ancient that nobody knows for sure who 'invented' it. Four thousand years ago – possibly more – the early spiritual seekers of northern India began to formulate meditation and austerity practices to help achieve and maintain a balanced existence. For centuries these teachings were passed down from gurus or priests to pupils, and because this was largely done by word of mouth, we have only limited information as to what these practices were, and how they evolved. However, a 20th-century discovery of artefacts from around that time caused great excitement. Archaeologists excavating the ruins of an early Indian civilisation that flourished in the Indus Valley in around 2,000BCE found small clay seals depicting what looked like a regal figure sitting cross-legged with the soles of the feet pressed together. Could this be a meditation pose? We don't know – but the possibility is tantalising.

The first millennium BCE marked a period of high sophistication and comfort in India – great cities started to emerge and ideas began to be exchanged along flourishing trade routes. People had risen above basic subsistence and had the leisure to ponder questions such as: 'Is there more to life than the endless cycle of birth and death? Is there some higher force at work, and how do I find out more?'

Those who wanted to devote serious energy to exploring the 'who am I? why am I here?' conundrum turned their backs on the daily grind to live a life of intense contemplation in forests and caves. Being a renunciate was not for the fainthearted – the effort involved in austerities such as fasting, standing for days on one leg, or lifelong silence was intense. The pay-off, however, was believed to be an inner fire (*tapas*) which would destroy ignorance and reveal the answers to life's big questions. We have written texts from this time that tell us that there was an ongoing debate between the ascetics and ordinary householders as to whose life was better. 'This is still a valid question for us in our practice today,' says yoga historian and former monk Carlos Pomeda. 'How are we going to integrate yoga into our daily lives when there is a conflict between the two?' Different traditions would go on to offer different answers, but they all had one thing in common, says Pomeda, 'that yoga is a practice that you do to solve your existential dilemma'.

So it was in this context that the yogic tradition – which is not one but many continuously overlapping streams of thought – grew. Around the 8th century BCE, yoga was referred to in writings known as *The Upanishads*. These show a shift away from rituals and sacrifices to a more sophisticated search for the inner self. The word 'yoga' is used to describe the 'restraint of the senses' – looking inside ourselves for answers.

The Upanishads put forward the idea that we could experience spiritual liberation in our lifetime. The divine (*Brahman*) was something within us; we had just lost sight of it, and the challenge was to find it again. Buddhism and Jainism, which also developed around that time, had their own yogic elements such as the idea of karma (action bearing fruit), meditation, and ethical behaviours. All these traditions would influence one another over the centuries.

So what does yoga mean? It is often translated as 'union' (for which its Sanskrit root '*yuj*' – yoke – is often invoked as evidence). But it's more accurate to define it as 'an application of means or a method', says Pomeda, 'yoking ourselves to practices that cultivate our highest awareness'. Yoga is both the means and the goal of an inner journey of self-discovery.

Back to the history books. Yoga, up to the era of *The Upanishads*, was largely a male tradition dominated by the priests and the renunciates; not particularly practical if you had a job and a family. But then a revolution happened. Around the 3rd to the 2nd century BCE, one text – *The Bhagavad Gita* ('Song of the Lord') – reflected a change in who yoga was for. The *Gita* was a philosophical poem which would become a favourite of Indian political leader

Different traditions all had one thing in common – yoga is a practice you do to solve your existential dilemma.

Mahatma Gandhi and admired by thinkers such as Albert Einstein, Aldous Huxley and Dr Albert Schweitzer. Indeed it is still studied by schoolchildren in India for its debates between right and wrong. The *Gita* (right) offered a choice of yoga paths to suit all lifestyles and preferences – no cave-dwelling required. People could choose from three types of yoga – *bhakti* yoga (the path of devotion and worship), *jnana* yoga (the path of knowledge through studying philosophical texts) or *karma* yoga (the path of skilful action). Now, everyone had the wherewithal to access the inner wisdom that the early ascetics were after. But we're not talking about the 'pick and mix' yoga schools such as Iyengar yoga and Ashtanga on offer in centres today. Downward facing dog and triangle pose were still several lifetimes away. Yoga – whichever path you chose – was still a collection of mind/spirit practices.

In the centuries that followed, yoga masters began to compose their ideas into systems. One in particular, a yogi and scholar called Patanjali who lived around 200CE, synthesised these traditions in *The Yoga Sutras*. This is still a must-read text for anyone looking to deepen their yoga practice. These 196 aphorisms define yoga as a point beyond meditation called '*samadhi*', a state of super-awareness where all ignorance and suffering dissolve and we just 'are'. Yoga, says Patanjali, is where mental chatter ceases, the mind is totally still, and our true nature becomes evident.

We'd like to think that most yoga teachers today have a well-thumbed copy of the *Sutras* (meaning 'threads') in order to draw on its teachings, particularly the 'eight-limbed path', which Patanjali outlines. Seven of these eight elements (see page 18) – which include restraints on behaviour as well as yoga postures, breathing and meditation – are intended to be practised together to create the right conditions to experience the eighth limb – *samadhi*. *Asana* (postures) is one of those limbs, and in Patanjali's time it meant only meditation postures. Interestingly, given that *asana* is the form in which most of us practise yoga today, Patanjali tells us very little about it. He says that our *asana* (meaning 'seat') should be steady (*sthira*) and joyful (*sukham*)[1] so that we can sit for meditation without fidgeting or distraction. Patanjali's yoga – which

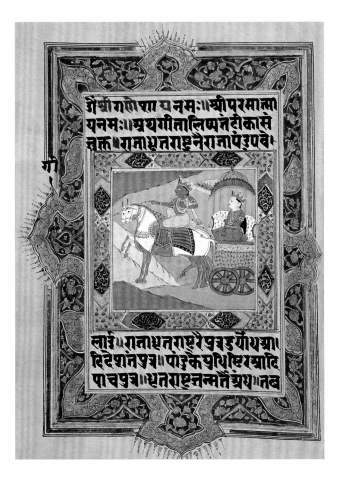

he calls *raja* yoga (meaning 'royal', denoting its supreme status) – gives us strategies to tame the mind and resist its emotional and psychological tangents.

WHERE'S MY DOWNWARD FACING DOG?

If Patanjali is telling us that *asana* is just about sitting in meditation, how did the *asanas* as we know them today become part of the yoga tradition?

At the time of Patanjali, the human body was not part of the spiritual quest. It was thought of as essentially impure – something best transcended. Patanjali did point out that a sick body wasn't conducive to *raja* yoga (if you are bugged by aches and pains, meditation is probably the last thing on your mind), but he didn't go into ways of staying healthy. However, tantric philosophy, which flourished around 8CE, placed the body centre stage in the spiritual journey. The body – not just the mind – could be purified to become a place where enlightenment happened. Tantra has been misunderstood as an 'anything goes' philosophy, says Pomeda, whereas in fact it's about using all that is available to us for our spiritual growth.

The tantrists gave us a detailed map of the subtle body – describing channels (*nadis*) through which vital energy known as *prana* flows and energy centres (chakras) where the channels meet. The goal of tantric practices (which include mantra, meditation, *pranayama* – or yoga breathing – and the use of specific herbs and internal cleansing practices called *kriyas*) was the expansion of consciousness in order to access the deepest levels of being. A dormant reservoir of vital energy known as *kundalini* (meaning 'coiled one') at the base of the spine could be awakened and directed up to the third-eye centre – a point between the eyebrows (*ajna* chakra) said to be the seat of wisdom. On its journey, it would purify the body – physically, mentally and emotionally – and, on arrival, consciousness would expand and all would be revealed. Tantra literally

means a tool ('*tra*') for expansion ('*tan*').

The tantrists laid the foundations for hatha yoga, a system whose physical aspect gives us many of the postures we do today. If you pick up *The Hatha Yoga Pradipika* ('Light on Hatha Yoga'), the 15th-century text by the sage Swatmarama, you may well come across things you recognise from your own practice, such as *gomukhasana* (cow face pose, page 158), *savasana* (corpse pose, page 40), the *bandhas* (page 170), and *pranayamas* such as *nadi shodhana* (alternate nostril breathing, page 168). You'll also find internal cleansing techniques, such as nasal cleaning (*neti*).

Hatha means 'forceful', reflecting the fact that it was tough work; raising *kundalini* didn't happen without dedicated effort. (Hatha also has the symbolic meaning derived from its Sanskrit components *ha*, 'sun', and *tha*, 'moon', symbolising opposites – passive and active, female and male energy – coming together in balance). But while the perfect body was a key feature of hatha

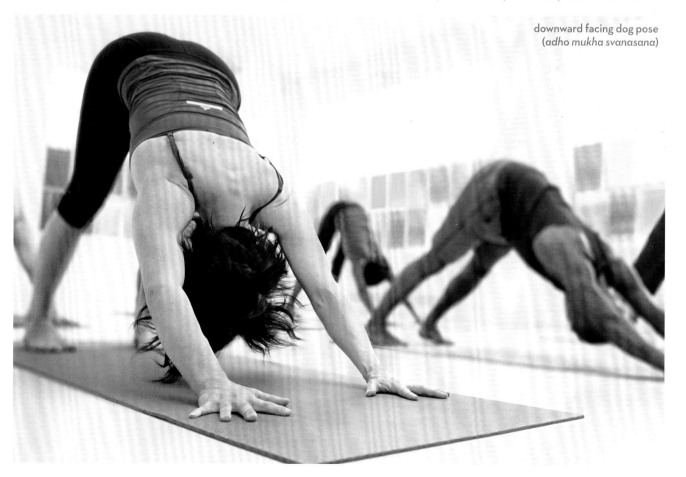

downward facing dog pose
(*adho mukha svanasana*)

yoga, it certainly wasn't an end in itself. If the body was free from impurities and blockages, prana could flow freely. The *Pradipika* spells out clearly that hatha yoga is the stairway to meditation where higher states of consciousness can be accessed. The yoga of Patanjali, as well as tantra and hatha, are three of the main philosophical currents through which the yoga tradition comes to us today.

There's one more philosophical system to mention and that's Advaita Vedanta. With its roots in *The Upanishads*, Advaita Vedanta emerged around the same time as tantra, but came to prominence in the late 19th century as one of the first yogic streams to make a major impact in the West. Its central theme is the 'oneness' of being – that we are all made up of the same energy and part of the same consciousness. Advaita translates as non-dual, meaning that humans and the divine are not separate entities. We all have that divine spark within us; we don't need to look outside ourselves for answers.

The 19th-century ambassador of Advaita Vedanta was a young, educated Hindu monk, Swami Vivekananda, who, in 1893, was asked to speak at the World Parliament of Religions in Chicago. He received a standing ovation from the 4,000-strong crowd for his message of tolerance and acceptance among all religions. His ideal of religion, he said, was becoming 'harmoniously balanced in love, work, wisdom and concentration... and this religion is attained by what we in India call yoga – union.'[2] Before his death in 1902 aged 39 he became an in-demand public speaker and was said to have introduced American oil tycoon John D Rockefeller to the idea of philanthropy.

This doesn't mean that yoga is a religion – it's not asking us to believe in anything outside ourselves. But it does mean that it can be a profoundly spiritual practice. If we go back to *The Upanishads*, we find the revolutionary idea that the absolute (*Brahman*) of which we are all part can be a personal god (*isvara*). It is a concept also expressed in the *Gita* and in the *bhakti* yoga devotional tradition, around the 5th century CE. Yoga is accepting of and compatible with all religions, yet not a religion in itself.

At the time that Vivekananda was spreading the

yogic word abroad, a five-year-old boy from the Indian state of Mysore was studying *The Yoga Sutras*. Tirumalai Krishnamacharya (1888–1989) was said to be descended from a revered 9th-century yogi and in 1916 went to study with one of the few remaining hatha yoga masters in Tibet. He returned to Mysore in 1924 and, while working as a teacher at the Sanskrit college there, came to the attention of the king of Mysore, a strong supporter of the traditional Indian arts. The king invited Krishnamacharya to set up a yoga school in the palace gymnasium and sponsored him to carry out yoga demonstrations all over India. Krishnamacharya developed a demanding *asana*-based form of yoga called 'vinyasa'. It is very likely that vinyasa was influenced by other sports going on in the gymnasium at the time, such as gymnastics and Indian wrestling. Later, Krishnamacharya became known as a great healer of illnesses through yoga.

He never came to the West, but his influence as a teacher of teachers can still be felt worldwide. Chances are that your teacher trained in the tradition of one of his main pupils – BKS Iyengar (known for his alignment-based and therapeutic approach), Sri K Pattabhi Jois (founder of Ashtanga yoga) and Krishnamacharya's son TKV Desikachar (who developed a healing approach tailored to each individual called viniyoga). As international travel improved in the second half of the 20th century all three of his pupils travelled widely – as did Krishnamacharya's first female pupil, Russian émigrée Indra Devi. In 1947 she brought yoga to Hollywood, teaching Greta Garbo, Gloria Swanson and Marilyn Monroe and eventually established several yoga centres in Argentina.

Other teachers too had a hand in yoga's journey to the West at that time. Swami Vishnudevananda brought Sivananda yoga (see page 29) to San Francisco in the 1950s. There are now Sivananda centres all over the globe. The Maharishi Mahesh Yogi – best known as the Beatles' guru and teacher of Californian wellbeing expert Deepak Chopra – developed Transcendental Meditation, a technique for stilling the mind. Meanwhile, devout Sikh Yogi Bhajan, who served in the Indian government, brought Kundalini yoga to California in 1969. He reached out to the prevalent

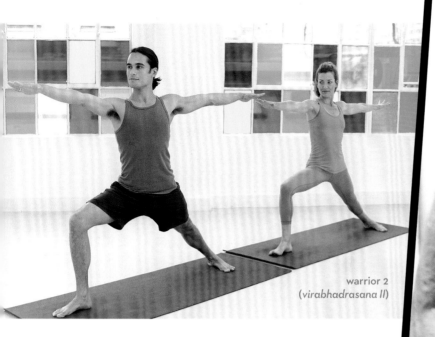

warrior 2
(*virabhadrasana II*)

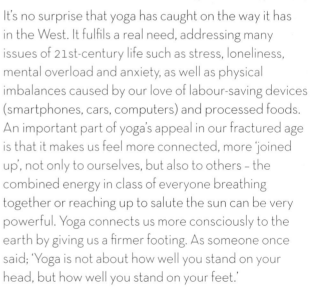

'Yoga is not about how well you stand on your head, but how well you stand on your feet.'

youth drug culture, offering an alternative 'inner euphoria' through yoga. Practitioners of the style say it can be effective at combating addiction.

WHAT DOES 'YOGA' MEAN NOW?

Given how yoga has morphed over 4,000 years, is there any simple answer to the question 'what is yoga'?

On one level it's a physical practice that makes us feel stronger, more flexible, less stressed, and generally better in ourselves. On another level, it's a set of spiritual attitudes and techniques to help us get to know who we are. Whatever our reasons for doing our practice, it quickly becomes apparent that after class we feel a little more calm, a little more 'in our body', with perhaps a better perspective of what's going on in our life. And this feeling gradually starts to inform everything we do.

Do we need to know its history? Actually, no. But it's reassuring hear that there are 4,000 years of research and development behind it. How many other exercise or wellbeing practices can say that?

It's no surprise that yoga has caught on the way it has in the West. It fulfils a real need, addressing many issues of 21st-century life such as stress, loneliness, mental overload and anxiety, as well as physical imbalances caused by our love of labour-saving devices (smartphones, cars, computers) and processed foods. An important part of yoga's appeal in our fractured age is that it makes us feel more connected, more 'joined up', not only to ourselves, but also to others – the combined energy in class of everyone breathing together or reaching up to salute the sun can be very powerful. Yoga connects us more consciously to the earth by giving us a firmer footing. As someone once said; 'Yoga is not about how well you stand on your head, but how well you stand on your feet.'

So every time you step on a yoga mat you connect to an evolving and powerful ancient tradition. Yoga is the ultimate, time-honoured method of self-improvement inside and out. There are many ways of getting there. Whatever your build, age, gender, religion or lifestyle, there is a type of yoga to suit your body and mind.

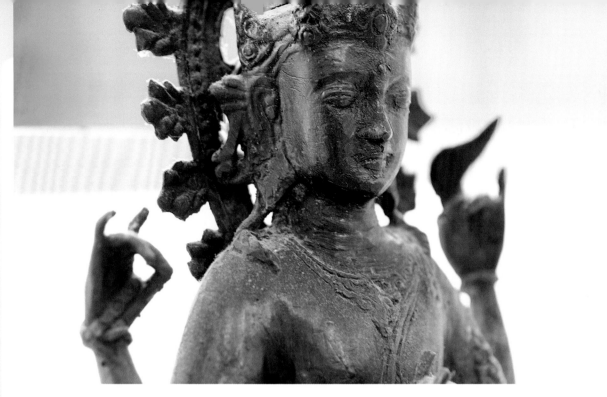

the eight limbs of yoga

If you are interested in yoga as more than just a physical exercise, the first concepts of yoga philosophy that you are likely to come across are the 'eight limbs'. If you have done yoga before, you will have practised at least one of these limbs – *asana* (posture), and maybe even also *pranayama* (breathing exercises) or *dhyana* (meditation).

These eight limbs or components of yoga were handed down by the Indian sage Patanjali in *The Yoga Sutras*, composed around 2,000 years ago. The *Sutras* are a practical guide to help us towards the goal of yoga – restraining the activities of the mind in order to experience a point beyond meditation called 'samadhi'. *Samadhi* is a state where we are totally absorbed in our essential Self and this, in turn, leads to liberation.

Patanjali called his eight-fold path Ashtanga yoga. 'Ashta' means eight, 'anga' means limbs (not to be confused with the dynamic hatha yoga practice of the same name). 'His advice is practical rather than moral,'

says yoga teacher Lucy May Constantini, who explains the eight limbs, below. 'If we want to know the Self, Patanjali gives us a ladder of spiritual practice – the eight limbs – to help structure our approach. These eight limbs do not need to be practised in any particular order but rather in response to the needs of each individual.'

1. YAMA – guidelines for behaviour

Patanjali tells us that restraint is a way to achieve the goal of yoga. The *yamas* are ways of reining in our behaviour – and include not stealing, being truthful, not harming, sexual continence and avoiding greed.

2. NIYAMA – practices to observe

These are purity, contentment, austerities, self-study and devotion to God.

Patanjali does not have a moral agenda with *yama* and *niyama*. They are simply ways of living to ensure that we are less likely to have disturbances in our mind and so can more easily achieve *samadhi* (meditative absorption, the eighth limb). If we spend our time lying, stealing, killing and sleeping around, we are not likely to find quiet and focused meditation attainable.

3. ASANA – posture

In Patanjali's time, this referred to a firm and comfortable posture for meditation. It has since developed into what most people refer to as 'yoga': a full hatha yoga practice to maintain a healthy body and calm the mind.

4. PRANAYAMA – controlling the breath

We control the breath, says Patanjali, to strengthen our understanding of the nature of the Self. Through certain *pranayama* practices 'the veil over the inner light is destroyed/And the mind becomes fit for *dharana*' (concentration, the sixth limb).[1]

Common techniques such as *ujjayi* breath and alternate nostril breathing, breath of fire and so on are thought to be later developments made possible by the advent of tantra in the 8th century. These days we also practise *pranayama* to balance the energy pathways (*nadis*) and to still the mind.

5. PRATYAHARA – drawing the senses inwards

Patanjali defines *pratyahara* as withdrawing the senses from external objects in order gain supreme mastery over the senses.[2] Practising *pratyahara* quietens and strengthens the mind, which makes *samadhi* possible.

Pratyahara is the opposite of the constant sensory bombardment of the modern world – the ping of an email, the invasiveness of an advertisement, the smell of your favourite perfume, the background music in a shop – all of which draw our attention outwards. For meditation, we need to channel our attention the other way – inwards. So when we are in a yoga class and we remember to focus on our own breath and body rather than looking around the room, we're starting to cultivate *pratyahara*.

6. DHARANA – concentration

This means directing our attention to one place. Common points of focus can include the breath, the space between the breaths or an internalised mantra – all concentration practices that lead to meditation. Patanjali was not dogmatic about what your point of focus should be. In theory you can focus on a tiddlywink if that gets you to *samadhi*.

7. DHYANA – meditation

Patanjali defines *dhyana* as prolonging the contemplation of the one point chosen in *dharana*. So where *dharana* teaches us to concentrate, *dhyana* strengthens our focus so it can become firm enough to perceive the Self.

For Patanjali, meditation means holding our attention on one point. There are hundreds of meditation techniques now practised.

8. SAMADHI – meditative absorption in the Self

By 'absorption' we mean that all of our attention is in the experience of *samadhi*. There's no brain activity left to think about it, comment on it or complain about our legs going to sleep or to wonder how much longer we have to sit here in meditation.

What is meant by the Self is a little trickier for us in a Western context. Earlier ideas in *The Upanishads* described the nature of the Self as pure being, pure consciousness and pure bliss (*saccidananda*). But as Patanjali was an ascetic, bliss wasn't top of his agenda. He was more interested in *samadhi* as a route to liberation (*kaivalya*) from the cycle of birth and death. This idea of 'liberation' may seem remote to us coming to yoga in the West and we may not share a world view that encompasses rebirth and liberation. But that doesn't mean that we can't enjoy the benefits of the yogic path Patanjali gives us.

At the very least, through the practices of yoga, our goal can be to find liberation from the parts of ourselves that hold us back from a calm, centred, blissful state.

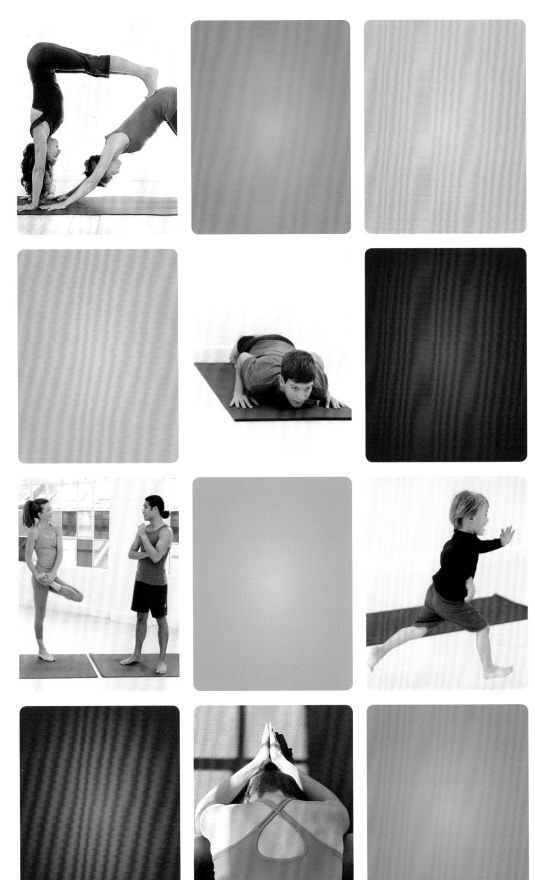
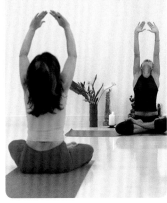
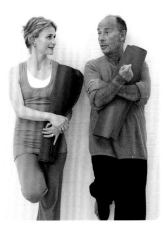
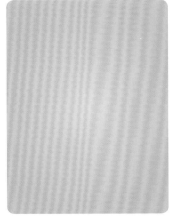
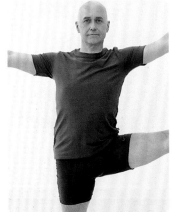

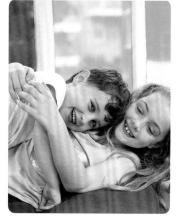
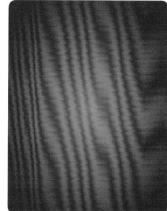
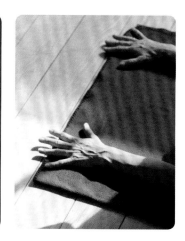

getting started

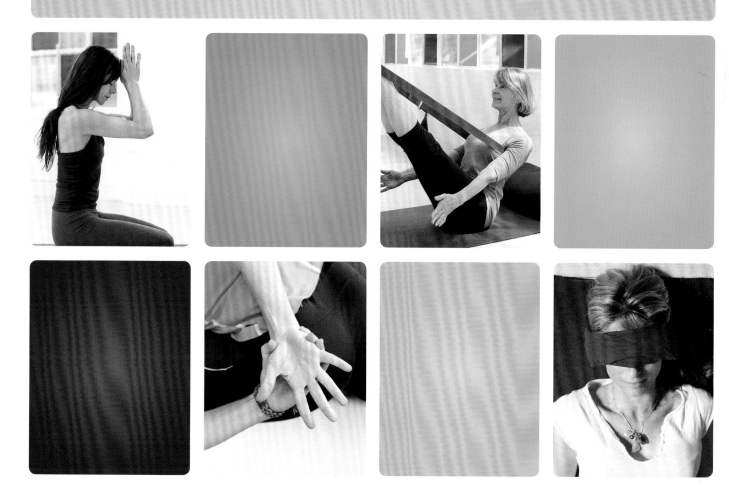

finding your yoga fit

Taking your first step on to the mat is an exciting new beginning. Whichever style you choose, building a solid foundation with the best possible teacher is the most important part of your practice

BY VICTORIA WOODHALL

Yoga is for everyone: it doesn't matter how old (or young) you are, how fit or unfit, or whether you are flexible or not – in fact, if you are stiff, you are the perfect candidate for yoga. If you have tight shoulders/back/hips, if you are overweight or under stress, yoga will help greatly. Even naturally flexible people can benefit in gaining strength and stability that they may lack.

When you are new to class (and even when you're not) it's easy to fall into the trap of comparing yourself with the bendy person at the front, who seems to be able to do everything without props and without breaking into a sweat. But apart from possibly being demoralising, looking at someone else's mat stops us from listening to what's going on in our own body. The mind loves to distract us, but try not to let what others are doing steal your attention. Yoga is your own personal journey.

SO MANY STYLES, SO MANY FANCY NAMES...

But which one is right for you? First ask yourself what you would like from your class. Maybe it's to de-stress or work out, relax, lose weight, stretch or tone, to follow a meditative or spiritual practice – or any combination of these.

Each style has its own unique emphasis. Some are at the more spiritual end of the spectrum and may begin with chanting. Others don't even feature so much as an 'Om'. Some move in a continuous flow, while others allow you to stop and ask questions. Some are practised with uplifting music, others in a quiet, candlelit space.

In the beginning it may be helpful to stick with one teacher or style. This will help to avoid confusion, as poses may be taught differently across different styles. Even within some methods, the pace and focus can vary depending on who's teaching and the level of the class. To find out the specifics, check out the teacher's website or talk to the front-of-house staff at your yoga centre. On the following pages you will find a list of the most common styles practised today. For a more detailed explanation of some of these see the 'styles in focus' chapter (page 44).

Always inform your teacher if you are pregnant or have any injuries, and if you have any medical conditions, please check with your doctor before starting yoga.

AcroYoga

Blending acrobatics, yoga and Thai massage, AcroYoga is mainly done in pairs with the emphasis on cultivating trust and playfulness. Its USP is 'flying', where one student lies down and acts as the 'base' and balances the other (the 'flier') either in an active pose such as bow, or a passive one such as a supported inversion where the flier hangs loosely upside down over the base. Although it can be physically challenging, there are entry points for beginners, who focus on solo *asana* sequences to prepare them for 'flying'.

Each style has its own unique emphasis. Some are at the more spiritual end of the spectrum and may begin with chanting. Others don't even feature so much as an 'Om'.

triangle pose (*trikonasana*)

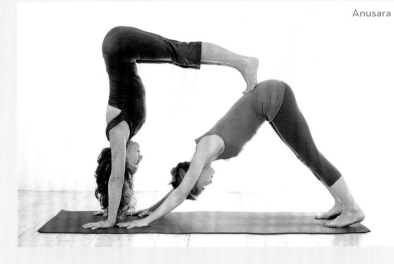
Anusara

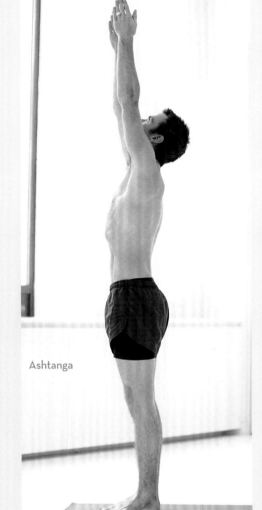
Ashtanga

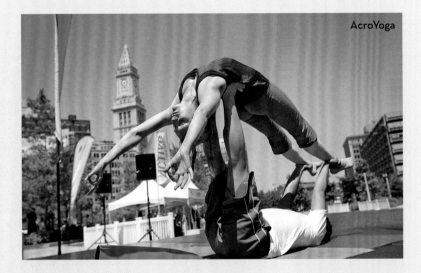
AcroYoga

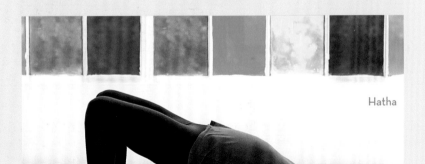
Hatha

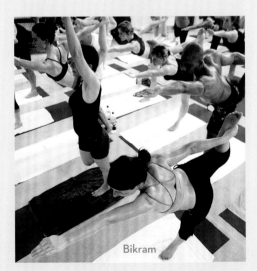
Bikram

Anusara

Anusara means 'flowing with grace' and following your heart. The emphasis is on opening the heart space both physically – by working on the chest, shoulders and upper back – as well as emotionally by connecting with your sense of playfulness and joy. It is one of the fastest-growing yoga styles today and is an upbeat yet physically demanding approach to hatha yoga with strong philosophical and alignment principles. In keeping with the heart theme, poses are instructed from the inside out – focusing on what they feel like rather than how they look.

Ashtanga

A physically demanding, flowing style requiring a certain level of fitness and readiness to sweat. Postures are held for a relatively short time and practised in a set sequence. The emphasis is on internal 'locks' (*bandhas*), fixing the gaze (*drsti*) and powerful breath (*ujjayi*).

It takes its name from the eight-fold philosophical path set out by Patanjali in *The Yoga Sutras* ('*ashta*' means eight; '*anga*' means limb). Ashtanga yoga as we know it today is a system of postures developed by the late Sri T Krishnamacharya and his pupil Pattabhi Jois in the 1930s. There are six sequences; most yoga classes will teach only the first – the primary series.

Bikram

A sequence of 26 postures and two breathing exercises done twice over in a carpeted, mirrored studio heated to 105 °F (40.5 °C) to make the muscles more flexible. There's a lot of sweating, so classes are very humid. Its colourful founder Bikram Choudhury was four-times National India Yoga Champion and is now based in Los Angeles. Postures are interspersed by brief relaxation. Because of the heat students are instructed to drink water during class.

Dynamic yoga

More of a generic term than a discrete style, 'dynamic' is a movement-based way of practising yoga *asana*, often involving sun salutations and flowing sequences, as opposed to styles such as Iyengar yoga, in which postures are held for longer.

Forrest yoga

An intensely physical and internally focused practice for healing physical and emotional pain, pioneered by Ana T Forrest. The style is founded on four pillars: breath, strength, integrity (tailoring poses to individual physical and emotional needs) and spirit (defined in the Native American sense as 'that which moves in all things'), accessed through breath and *asana* practice.

Hatha yoga

A general term for 'yoga' combining physical poses, breathing techniques and meditation. Classes can vary widely and many teachers have developed their own style within the hatha tradition to reflect their preferred practice.

Insight yoga

A style of yoga combining insights from the yogic, Taoist and Buddhist traditions formulated by Sarah Powers, founder (with her husband Ty) of the Insight Yoga Institute in California. Insight yoga combines both passive (Yin yoga, see page 29) and dynamic flow (*yang*) practice based on the idea that this enhances all our bodily tissues and integrates the *yin* and *yang* sides of our personalities and moods.

Integrative Yoga Therapeutics™

Developed by Boston-based clinical psychologist, yoga teacher and yoga therapist Bo Forbes, this method is an integration of yoga, psychology and science for the purpose of healing to address issues such as physical injuries, anxiety, depression, insomnia, chronic pain, immune disorders – and also for performance enhancement.

Iyengar yoga

The Iyengar method is internationally respected for its detailed structural approach. Props may be used to aid correct alignment and to enable students – regardless of age or flexibility – to access the benefits of challenging postures and to progress at their own pace. BKS Iyengar (born 1918) has been one of yoga's chief modern global ambassadors with a direct lineage to the ancient teachings via his brother-in-law

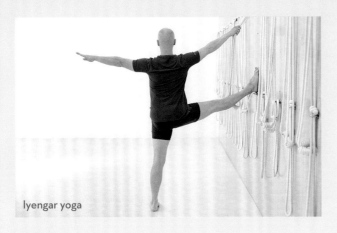
Iyengar yoga

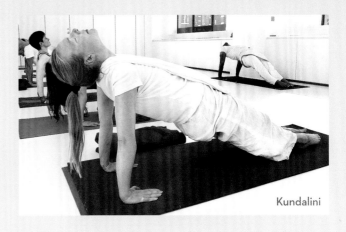
Kundalini

Sri T Krishnamacharya. He runs the Ramamani Iyengar Memorial Yoga Institute in Pune, India, and is known for his success in using yoga to treat a wide range of medical conditions.

Jivamukti
A vinyasa-based method founded in New York by Sharon Gannon and David Life, featuring hands-on adjustments, *pranayama*, and chanting accompanied by music that enhances the 'focus of the month'. This focus can be anything from 'standing poses', to '*anahata* chakra' to 'fear' or a particular Yoga Sutra. For an extra fee, students can book an 'in-studio private' where they are adjusted by a dedicated teacher. Jivamukti means 'liberated while living'.

Kirtan
Kirtan refers to chanting, traditionally one of the main practices of yoga. Indian instruments such as the harmonium and drum accompany the chant while Sanskrit mantras are repeated in a call-and-response fashion, bringing about a stilling of the mind and an connection to our 'feeling" rather than 'thinking' state.

Kripalu
Kripalu emphasises the carrying-over of lessons from the yoga mat into everyday life. The premise is that the more we develop our self-knowledge and non-judgemental awareness (or witness consciousness), the better we can choose how to act on our thoughts and feelings and to find stillness in difficult situations.

The Kripalu Institute for Extraordinary Living runs a number of research programmes into the mental and physical benefits of yoga with Harvard Medical School.

Kundalini
Kundalini uses five tenets of yogic science – mantra, *pranayama*, *mudra*, meditation plus rhythmic and static *asana* to target the glandular and central nervous systems in order to balance body chemisty. Instructors (usually wearing white, signifiying neutrality and impartiality) teach from thousands of *kriyas* – sequences with specific effects such as aiding digestion or metabolic balance. These may involve rapid, repetitive movements, demanding considerable mental stamina. Most classes are 'open' level (see page 31) and each student works within their range. The emphasis is less on dynamic stretching, more on core strength and physical/mental cleansing.

Mysore-style Ashtanga
Early-morning Ashtanga yoga as taught in Mysore, India, by the late Sri K Pattabhi Jois, the originator of Ashtanga yoga. Yoga centres usually offer a two-to-three-hour window from about 6am where you can practise the Ashtanga primary series (or beyond) at your own pace, supervised and adjusted by a teacher.

Never-too-late yoga
A class for those who feel they have passed a point of no return for yoga, this style is designed to accommodate anyone who wants an entry point to the

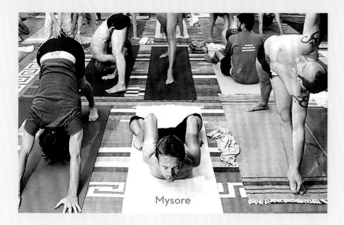

Mysore

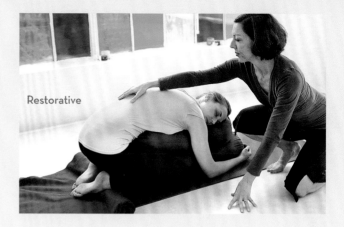

Restorative

practice that they wrongly think is accessible only to the young and fit. The teacher uses props to support people who are basically well but have restricted movement or require more personal attention. For seniors, restorative yoga and 'yoga gently' classes are also a suitable entry points.

OM yoga
A medium-paced, playful style of hatha yoga that combines flowing yoga *asanas*, precise attention to alignment and Buddhist mindfulness meditation. Founded by former dancer Cyndi Lee in New York, OM yoga has a strong teacher-training arm, including a special course on how to teach cancer survivors.

ParaYoga
ParaYoga (para meaning 'supreme' or 'highest'), founded by Rod Stryker, is an *asana*-based practice that also integrates other elements of traditional yoga: *pranayama*, *bandha*, *mudra*, visualisation, meditation, chanting, *kriya*, mantra, *kundalini*. Emphasis is on improving the quality of the individual's energy in order to improve quality of life.

Postnatal yoga/Mummy and Me
Postnatal yoga offers specialist teaching for strengthening the mind and body from 40 days after giving birth and the chance to breathe deeply and undo some of the tensions of carrying a baby. 'Mummy and Me' combines postnatal yoga with fun singing, dancing and movement for baby up to crawling.

Power yoga
A term used by some teachers of dynamic yoga, for example Baron Baptiste's Power Vinyasa Yoga.

Purna yoga
Purna yoga (*purna* meaning 'complete' or 'whole') teaches alignment-based *asana*, *pranayama* and heart-centred meditation as well as 'healthy living' classes, encompassing diet as well as yoga philosophy and its relationship to daily life. It was founded by former corporate lawyer Aadil Palkhivala, who trained with BKS Iyengar from the age of seven, and his wife, meditation and Kundalini master Savitri.

Remedial yoga
One-on-one sessions providing specific programmes for managing injuries and physical conditions. The teacher may also explain techniques to help students wishing to continue with their regular class to work safely around their injury or condition.

Restorative yoga
Designed for relaxation and rejuvenation and especially beneficial for nervous exhaustion, stress or 'information overload'. Poses are mostly done lying down and supported over bolsters using straps, blocks, eye-bags and blankets. Restorative yoga was pioneered by BKS Iyengar who developed it for those who were unable to do a more vigorous practice; it has been evolved more recently by Judith Hanson Lasater, who studied with him.

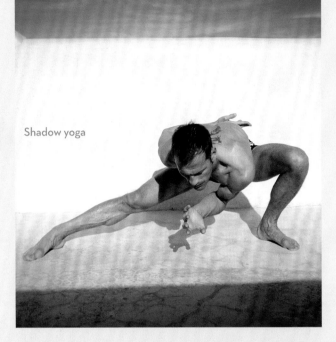

Shadow yoga

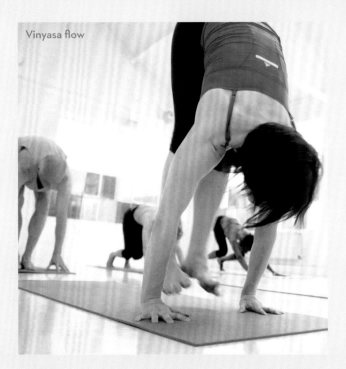

Vinyasa flow

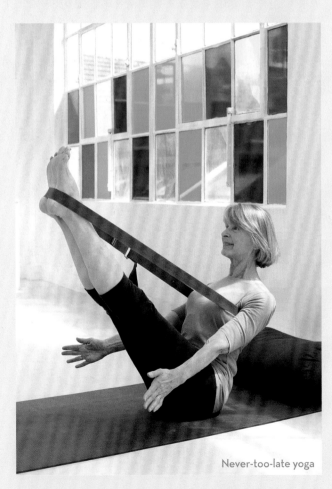

Never-too-late yoga

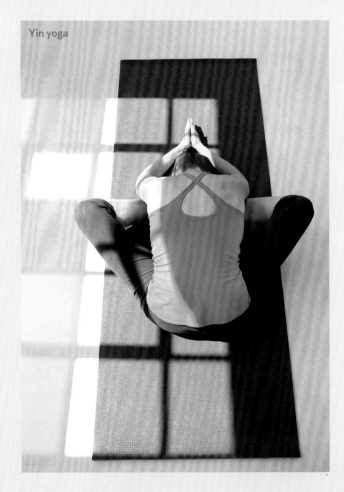

Yin yoga

Scaravelli-inspired yoga

This slow, subtle yet challenging style works with breath and gravity to release and extend the spine, re-educating it back to suppleness and health. Students focus on the sensations in their body from moment to moment, noticing physical and emotional tension and working with the intelligence of the spine to release it. Scaravelli is not a method as such, but an approach to practice inspired by Vanda Scaravelli (1908–1999), who crystallised her teachings in her 1991 book, *Awakening the Spine*.

Shadow yoga

A powerful, fluid practice founded by Zhander Remete, beginning with 'preludes' – sequences rather like a yogic/martial arts dance with yoga positions such as *chaturanga*, warrior stances and forward bends. These 'preludes' often move beyond the confines of the mat and prepare the body for other *asana* by first releasing mental and physical restrictions.

Sivananda yoga

A slow-paced sequence of 12 postures to open the energy channels and stimulate the chakras. Classes begin with chanting, breathing exercises (*prananyama*) and sun salutations immediately followed by strong inversions (headstand, shoulder stand, plough). These are modified for beginners. Its founder was Indian doctor-turned-monk Swami Sivananda (1887–1963) whose disciple Swami Vishnudevananda brought Sivananda's teachings to the West in 1957.

Yoga therapy

Specialist classes and one-to-ones for health conditions such as arthritis, asthma, cancer, diabetes, depression, high blood pressure, HIV and AIDS, lower back pain, ME, MS, sports injuries and menopause. The UK Yoga Biomedical Trust provides training in certain aspects of yoga therapy, holds directories of yoga therapists in the UK and researches yoga therapy. The International Association of Yoga Therapists in America holds an annual symposium on yoga research and publishes the *International Journal of Yoga Therapy*.

Vinyasa flow

A dynamic style of yoga in which movement is instructed with the breath (for example, 'inhale as you raise your arms, exhale as you fold forward'). Poses are held for a relatively short time and the flowing transition between postures is as important as the postures themselves. *Vinyasa* in Sanskrit means 'to place in a special way' and comes from the yogic technique of '*vinyasa krama*' – ordering your yoga practice intelligently so that each step is a step in the right direction towards your goal. Applied to *asana* practice, this means linking postures in such a way that each provides the groundwork for the next so that challenging poses are attempted once the body has been strengthened and opened safely.

Viniyoga

Viniyoga was developed by by TKV Desikachar (son of Sri T Krishnamacharya) as a one-to-one method of teaching, tailoring the yoga practice to the individual's needs and life stage. Gary Kraftsow, who trained with Desikachar, set up the American Viniyoga Institute in California and evolved the practice to include teaching in small groups. This gentle style lends itself to therapeutic use. The Viniyoga Therapist Training Program trains existing teachers in the therapeutic use of yoga for health conditions.

Yin yoga

Yin requires muscles to be soft and relaxed rather than engaged, in order to work into the deep connective tissues. Poses are held passively to load the ligaments safely so that the body responds by making them stronger and more pliant. Because it is also suggested that the body's energy channels run through the connective tissue, a Yin yoga practice increases energy distribution through these channels, a principle said to be similar to that of acupuncture. While this method – systematised and popularised by Paul Grilley – is passive, it brings up strong sensations and challenges students to be still and present in the face of discomfort, thereby encouraging mindfulness – non-judgemental awareness of the present moment.

what level am I?

beginner

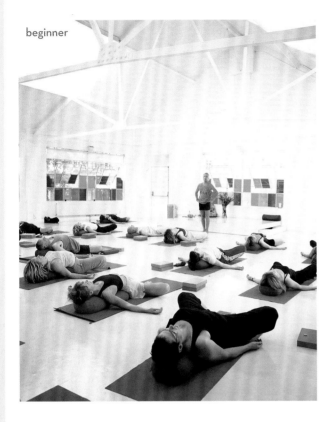

level 1

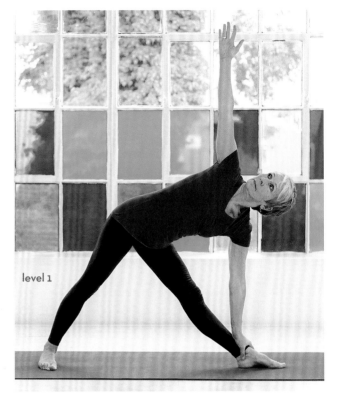

BEGINNER

A beginners' course – usually once a week over eight weeks – is a good introduction. You will be discovering yoga in a safe, fun space, learning the basics of breathing, movement and posture. The practice builds week by week.

Spend as much time as you need at beginner level. You can even take several beginners' courses. The time you spend here establishes the foundations of your practice.

If a course doesn't fit your timetable, Level 1 and Open Level classes are also suitable. Likewise 'yoga gently' and restorative classes, which are at the gentler end of the yoga spectrum, allowing beginners to integrate with ease.

In your first few yoga classes it is normal to be a little confused. In the course of your day no one tells you what to do with your right hip, your left shoulder blade or the crown of your head. In dynamic styles, this so-called 'proprioception' can be more challenging initially, since you need to find your body parts more quickly. But if you felt good afterwards, don't worry about whether or not you did it correctly. Enjoy the fact that no matter how hard it was, you were so engaged with the challenge that, for an hour or so, you weren't thinking about your to-do list.

LEVEL 1

These classes are aimed at complete beginners, those in the initial stages of yoga practice or those seeking a gentler practice. Many experienced students take Level 1 and Open Level classes out of choice, as working with the fundamentals of yoga practice is challenging as well as refreshing.

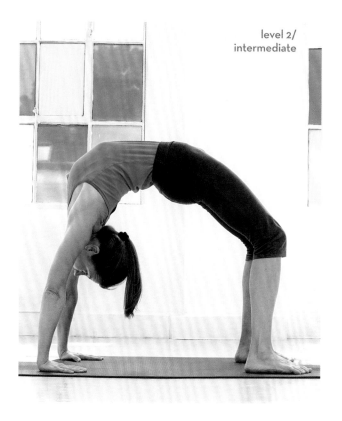

level 2/
intermediate

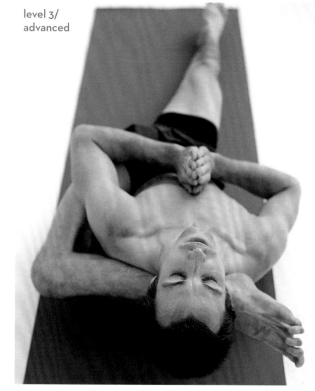

level 3/
advanced

OPEN LEVEL

The teacher adapts the class according to the students. In this mixed-ability class it might be tempting for beginners to try to keep up with long-term practitioners. Do what you can without straining. You'll go further if you work from where you are, not from where you think you should be.

LEVEL 2/INTERMEDIATE

Here the teacher works on a deeper physical and psychological level, introducing more challenging *asanas* ('postures'), sun salutation variations, inversions and backbends. These classes are not suitable for beginners. Knowledge of certain postures is assumed.

LEVEL 3/ADVANCED

A challenging class for more experienced practitioners, which assumes a good grounding in the principles of *asana* and breathing. For Level 3 Ashtanga classes, knowledge of the Ashtanga primary series is essential.

Don't be in a hurry to get to this level. Being an advanced yogi is not just about mastering difficult postures – although these can be fun and bring huge benefits. It's about the advanced level of awareness you bring to your practice. If, after a long time of trying, you finally manage the 'bind' in a difficult twist, that's progress indeed. But your challenge now is to find the same equanimity, the same even and steady breath that comes more easily in basic postures. This is where *asana* starts to become yoga in the traditional sense of finding stillness.

IF YOU'VE TRIED YOGA BEFORE AND DIDN'T LIKE IT...

What didn't you like? Too boring? Too full-on? Too new-agey? You didn't feel you were 'good' at it? Too uncomfortable? Too many intimidating-looking bendy people? Didn't like the teacher?

You're not the first to say so. Don't be put off yoga as a whole if the first class you try doesn't work. There are many types of ice cream, but you wouldn't write off the whole gamut of flavours because the first one you tasted was pistachio. Who knows, over time pistachio might even grow on you.

Finding the right class may take a little time at first. A high-achieving type-A personality might find a slow-paced class isn't enough of a challenge, bemoaning the fact that they 'hardly did anything' and where was the sweaty work-out? In that case, the advice would be to look for a dynamic class, such as vinyasa flow, Ashtanga or Jivamukti and in time to revisit that slower-paced class. It might in fact be what you need to balance out your go-go-go tendencies.

If you are the sort of person who prefers the subtlety, precision and calm of a slower-paced class, an hour of dynamic sun salutations and arm balances may generate more frustration than relaxation. You might prefer an Iyengar yoga or Sivananda class – or simply a different teacher whose pace matches yours. Yoga is the ultimate versatile practice as all forms of yoga lead to the same end – a calm, centred state of mind and more balanced energy.

WORKING YOUR EDGE

In many postures there will be a point at which you can't reach further or go any deeper. This is your edge. Your muscles are simply saying 'enough'. Trying to force your way through tension by jamming yourself into the pose can trigger the muscles to tighten further, because they are primed to prevent us from injuring ourselves. One of the fundamental principles of yoga is *ahimsa* – non-harming (see page 18). That includes not harming yourself. Remember to work into your edge mindfully and gradually and find an attitude of ease, a balance between effort and surrender where you can still breathe fully and your face is soft. You may find that the

muscles release a little and you can go deeper. Playing your edge is also a way of keeping your mind interested in the practice. If it wanders, that's the time when you are most susceptible to injury. Remember there is no such thing as 'good pain'. If you feel sharp or jabbing sensations, dizziness or if something simply doesn't feel quite right, stop immediately. If you want to rest, come into child's pose (page 157) or lie down on your back.

If you are unsure whether it's pain that you are feeling or the discomfort of tight muscles releasing, simply ease off. Yoga sharpens your powers of awareness and as you get to know your body better you will find it easier to distinguish between the sensation of working to your edge and doing something which could potentially cause injury.

BEING COMFORTABLE WITH DISCOMFORT

As you practise, it quickly becomes apparent that some poses come more easily to you than others. These vary from person to person, depending on how you have deployed your body over the years. If you are used to sitting cross-legged on the floor to watch TV, for example, your hips may naturally be more open than if you habitually use the sofa. If you are at your computer all day, the chest, shoulders, wrists, hands and thighs are likely to be fairly tight and feel stiff when you are asked to do poses that open or stretch them. If you are a cyclist, you will probably have strong but tight quads, hamstrings and glutes.

None of us likes to come up against our limitations, but this is the challenge that yoga throws at us. It puts our body through its full range of motion – forwards, backwards, sideways, upwards, downwards, twisting and opening – deploying muscles and joints that may not have received such full attention in long while. Props can help tension to release – there are no prizes (or benefits) in gritting your teeth and bearing it. Staying centred in the face of difficulty or discomfort can show us that we are not only physically but also mentally stronger than we think.

You might also find that a particular practice makes you feel emotionally uncomfortable – angry, frustrated or even weepy. As you work with your stiff back, for

Staying centred in the face of difficulty or discomfort can show us that we are not only physically but also mentally stronger than we think.

boat pose (*navasana*)

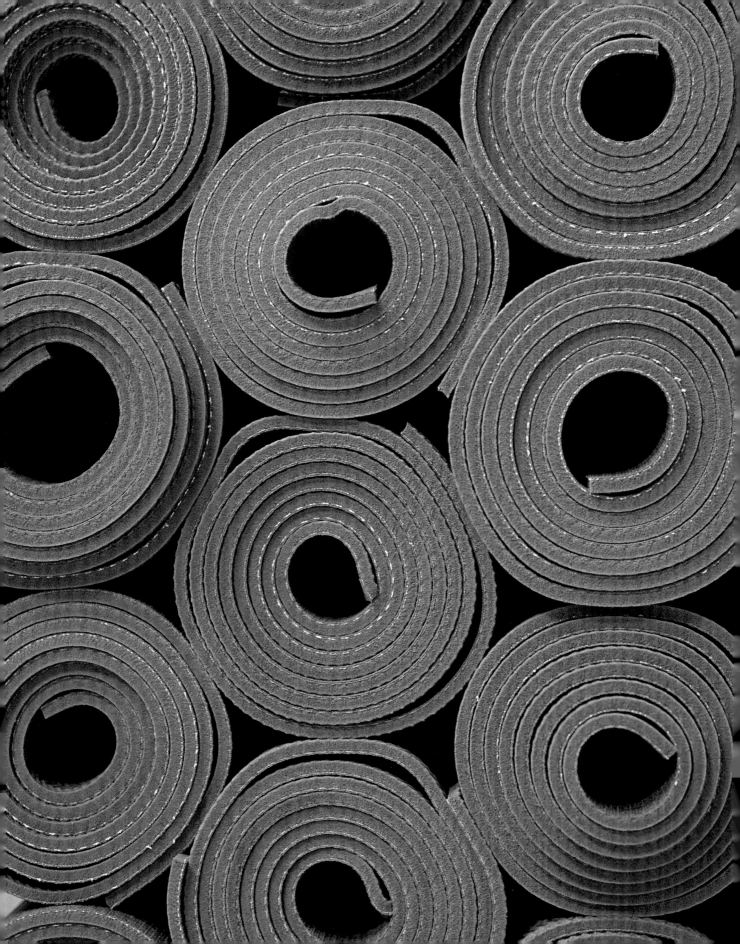

example, it could also bring up all the reasons why you are tight in the first place – the long hours you've been spending at your desk, or the heavy bags you have been carrying.

When doing postures we release physical tension, which may have built up for years. Sometimes this tension is linked to an emotion. For example, if we are deeply afraid of a situation, every time we come face to face with it, the body responds by curling in to protect itself. So when we start opening out the front of the body all the emotion that has become locked in begins to release. We can experience its release as the emotion itself, even though it is entirely out of context. Rather than being afraid or suppressing it,

see it as a letting-go of something that has simply been embedded physically. However, if it taps into something very troubling, please seek the help of a trained therapist.

For most of us, corpse pose (savasana) at the end of class is a chance for mind and body to settle and for the mind to turn inwards and rest.

At some point, everyone comes up against tension, whether it's physical, mental or emotional. But that's the great thing about yoga – it helps each of us where we need it. Coming face to face with the things that limit us is the first step to addressing them and to growing in our practice and as a person. This is the path to liberation that the ancient yogis talk about.

say it in Sanskrit!

Sanskrit is the ancient language of yoga. Some teachers will use Sanskrit terms, some will stick to their English equivalents, some will mix and match as we do in this book. Here are a few basic Sanskrit words you will come across:

Asana: Literally this means 'seat' but it's generally used to mean 'yoga posture'. In Sanskrit every posture name ends in *asana*. So, for example, triangle pose is *trikonasana* (*tri*=three, *kona*=angle, *asana*=posture). We use the term '*asana* practice' (doing postures) to distinguish it from the broader spectrum of what 'yoga' is. Chanting, meditation and studying philosophy, for instance, are also yoga practices. The catch-all term for physical yoga is 'hatha yoga'.

Om: Not a word as such, but a sound that is said to represent the

whole universe, which was created out of this sound. *Om* is composed of three separate sounds gliding into each other 'A-U-M' (aah, uuh, mmm) and chanting it helps to focus the mind and draw our attention inwards.

It is often used at the beginning of class to bring everyone together, and at the end to close the class. It is said that the most powerful part of this mantra is in the stillness that follows afterwards.

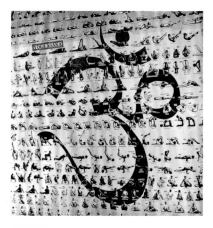

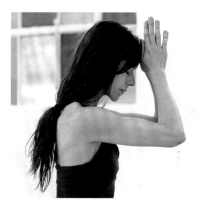

Namaste: Often used by teachers at the end of class, *namaste* means 'I bow to you' (*nama*=bow, *as*=I, *te*=you). It is a way of saying thank you and is often accompanied by the hands in prayer position (*anjali mudra*) and a little bow. Teachers may thank their students (and vice versa) for sharing their practice as well as their own teachers and gurus and the lineage through which the ancient teachings have been passed.

practice q + a

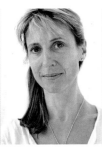

Not sure when and how to practise, what to wear on your feet or whether it's OK to skip the chanting? Jane Kersel answers frequently asked questions

Should I practise yoga if...

I have an injury?

If necessary, speak to your doctor first, and always tell your teacher at the beginning of class. He or she can offer you advice on modifying your practice. As a rule, sharp pain that feels 'electrical' is a warning sign and means you need to ease off.

If you have a long-standing injury, consider booking a one-on-one with a yoga therapist who has an in-depth knowledge of musculature and anatomy. Ask them to show you a few key techniques specific to your body that you can take with you into your regular class.

I have a cold?

If you're in the first stages of a cold, rest, stay warm and let your body heal. A fever is the body's natural way of killing off germs by heating them to a very high internal temperature. Adding yoga to your to-do list at this stage may only aggravate the system. Keep hydrated and eat lightly. If you have a viral infection, please don't spread germs by going to class.

If you're in the later stages of a cold with less acute symptoms, try a restorative class to help tight respiratory muscles (which may have been overworked because of a bad cough) to release as well as helping your nose to clear. Simple, light movement and gentle stretches help drain the lungs and will make you feel like you're on the mend.

I've been ill, have had surgery or am on medication?

There's no 'one size fits all' in yoga, therefore it's very important to be responsible for your own recovery. Talk to your doctor and relay their advice to your yoga teacher. If you are healing, keep the load off your body (as above).

Listen to your internal teacher too. There's a tendency nowadays to override how our bodies feel, to stay on the 'busy hamster wheel of life'. Yoga is also about mindfulness, so watch the part of you that might be trying to push yourself back into your daily routine and overdo things. Doing a hardcore dynamic practice when your body is telling you to slow down goes against the yogic idea of 'ahimsa' – non-harming (see The Eight Limbs of Yoga, page 18). Let the healing happen and use that as a time to try other practices of yoga, such as meditation.

I'm pregnant, can I go to my regular class?

Keeping going to your regular yoga teacher can feel like a must when pregnancy is causing so many other aspects of your life to change. But check first whether your teacher is trained in pregnancy yoga or has had children herself while she practised and is happy to continue teaching you with the correct modifications in a regular class. The onus is on you to ease up when you need to. Pregnancy is not a time to attempt new postures or push yourself.

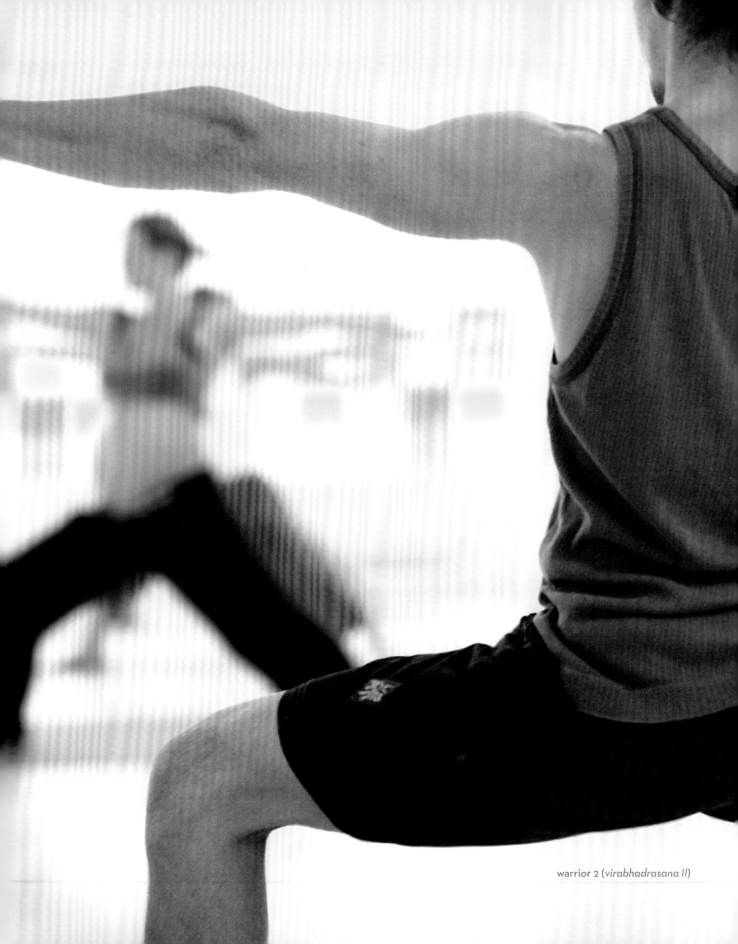

warrior 2 (*virabhadrasana II*)

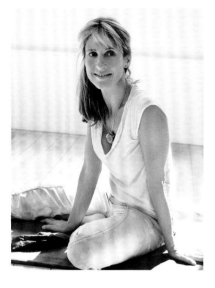

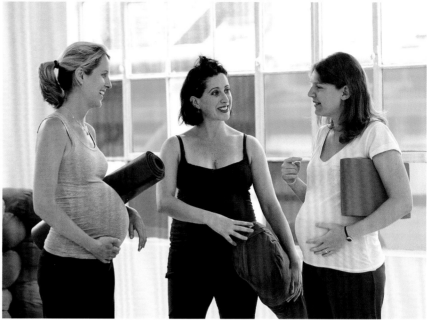

We practise barefoot in order to prevent slipping and to get the full use of the feet.

hand-to-foot pose (*padahastasana*)

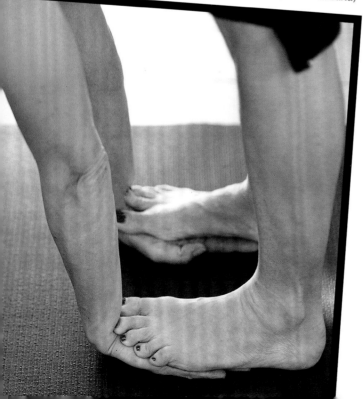

Generally, pregnant women should stand with the feet slightly wider than hip width apart, avoid closed twists which compress the abdomen and steer clear of strong backbends and lying on the abdomen. When forward bending, protect the lower back by bending the knees, making sure to allow space for the baby.

It is sometimes helpful to be around other pregnant women at this time, so try also a pregnancy yoga class. Certainly, if you have never done yoga before, this is where you need to start.

I've just eaten?

After a meal your energy will be directed towards digestion, so it wouldn't make sense to go to a yoga class afterwards, especially a dynamic one. A restorative class is less of a problem. Ideally, eat nothing two hours beforehand, and then only something light, and come well hydrated. If you're diabetic, take advice from your doctor and be aware that a hot class may have an effect on your medication.

As to whether you should drink water in class, remember that if you feel thirsty, you are already dehydrated, and that if you drink large amounts of water in class you'll feel it as you move around.

I'm wearing socks?

We practise barefoot in order to prevent slipping and to get the full use of our feet. The weight of the body falls entirely through the surface of the foot, so your teacher needs to be able to see how you place it. A firm contact with the earth through the foot also gives us the energetic sense of being grounded.

Washing your feet before class is a good habit to cultivate. It's respectful not just to yourself but also to others using the mat after you.

I'm overweight?

Yoga is for everyone, not just the lithe-and-bendy brigade. However, if you are overweight, a yoga class full of slim people can be daunting. Be brave and, rather than slipping away after class and not coming back, ask your teacher, 'What would you recommend to help me?'

Some of the more challenging poses such as rolling up into a shoulder stand may be a struggle, but everyone struggles with different postures for different reasons. A good teacher will help you or give the entire class an alternative pose to avoid singling anyone out.

Traditionally, standing poses such as mountain or chair are taught with feet together, but if you are overweight this may not be possible. Some teachers take the feet hip width apart, which may suit you better.

If you are coming to yoga to lose weight, there are a number of ways it can help. While a yoga class will not burn fat as effectively as, say, a 5km run, there's no reason why you shouldn't take up running and yoga.

Heated classes may bring more rapid weight loss, as heat not only raises the metabolic rate but also increases cardiovascular activity. There are various types of hot yoga, some of which use fan or radiator heat and others which use 'far infra-red' heat. The latter may help to release toxins at a deeper level. These are then expelled through sweat and urine.

Yoga doesn't necessarily have to be hot or 'power yoga' to initiate weight loss. Any yoga – even a regular meditation practice – is a way of establishing a deeper connection to your body and creating an internal space where you may begin to feel better about yourself on

Yoga doesn't necessarily have to be hot or 'power yoga' to initiate weight loss.

many levels. Once people let go of how they 'should' be, they often naturally start to lose weight. They lose the need to binge or comfort eat and generally crave healthier foods.

In becoming more mindful, you may find yourself more aware of the emotions that trigger overeating. With consciousness comes the possibility of change.

I'm self-conscious about chanting?

Chanting is usually done in Sanskrit, the ancient language of yoga, at the beginning and end of class. Not all styles incorporate it, but if they do, it's nothing to do with hitting the right note (or, for that matter, necessarily with religion – see page 40). Sound is an ancient yogic path called 'nada yoga' and can have a profound effect on the cells of the body. As they resonate, they are bathed in a healing sound wave. Try brahmari (humming bee breath, see page 71) and see how it makes a wonderful 'sound bath' for the brain, leaving it clearer, lighter, more energised.

Sound is a way of bypassing the conscious mind, of moving from thinking mode to feeling mode, creating a connection with the body. Repeating a phrase or sound helps focus your mind on one point; and the fact that you are not chanting in English means that you are less likely to 'go places' in your mind with the words. When the thinking mind is quiet we can start to access the subconscious levels of the mind where healing can happen.

You can also think of chanting as a way of connecting to the ancient teachings of yoga, in that you are accessing a sacred mantra which has been used for thousands of years.

If you would still prefer not to join in, you can enjoy the experience of the sounds by just sitting and letting the vibrations move through you in a healing way.

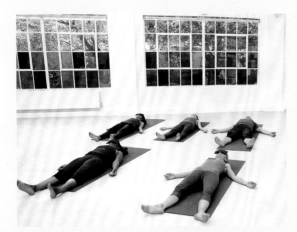

Why do we always do corpse pose?

Resting in corpse pose (*savasana*) for ten minutes or so at the end of a session works powerfully on many levels.

1. RELEASING. It releases the muscles and integrates the work you've done in class, before you go about the rest of your day.

2. HEALING. It is also a chance to drop from your thinking mind into your subconscious layers, where healing can happen.

3. REJUVENATING. Relaxing while awake is extremely beneficial for the nervous system (see restorative yoga page 76).

Although *savasana* seems so simple – it's only lying down, after all – some people find it extremely challenging. If you are worried that your life is crashing in, and you feel you've already spent too much time in the yoga class, coax yourself to stay for at least a few minutes and build up so that eventually you take the full time. Investing a few minutes of your time here gives you even more energy and capability to do what you need to do later.

I have my own religion?

While you will find elements of yoga philosophy in Hinduism, the practice itself is non-religious. You can do yoga and have your own faith, or none. Yoga is a way of creating the space and time to connect to what you truly believe in beyond all the patterns and conditioning of your upbringing or your social 'tribe'.

You might see a dancing Shiva statue or a meditating Buddha surrounded by candles and flowers at the front of the class or your teacher might lead a chant to specific deities. None of this seeks to impose a set of beliefs on you. It's a way of invoking the energy and attributes that the deity represents. Shiva, for example, is the god of yoga, often represented in his cosmic dance, crushing ignorance, surrounded by a ring of fire; Ganesh, the elephant deity, is said to be the remover of obstacles; Lakshmi is the goddess of happiness and abundance and a Buddha, the enlightened sage and great meditator, resonates calm and loving kindness.

I am naturally very flexible anyway?

Yoga isn't about flexibility alone, but also about strength, balance and integration of the joints. Flexibility needs strength and vice versa.

If you're naturally very bendy, you need to be mindful not to damage your joints by overstretching. Work on drawing the bones deep into their sockets. In tree pose, for example, it's easy for the standing leg to lean out (as it would if you were balancing a baby on your hip), causing the top of the thigh bone to press against the outer edge of the socket rather than integrating into it. A feeling of integration is what we should all look for in every pose, but hypermobile people especially.

Consider booking a one-on-one with a yoga therapist to advise you on the safest way to practise for your body.

I've just had a baby?

After a baby, you may feel in need of your yoga practice more than ever. If you are breastfeeding, you may be more rounded in the shoulders than usual or have a stiff neck. You may have heavy, swollen breasts which might make your back ache. Plus, it takes a few weeks to

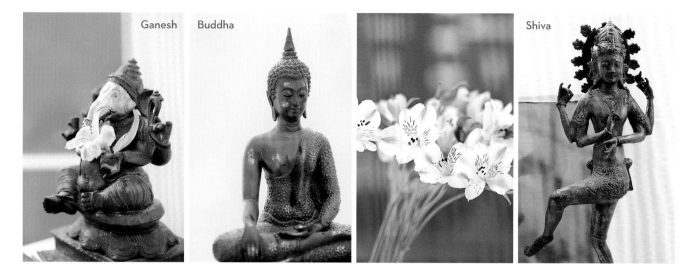

Ganesh   Buddha   Shiva

regulate your milk supply to the point at which it feels comfortable to exercise.

There will be extra stiffness and imbalance from sitting on your bottom more than you are used to, from carrying the baby and pushing a buggy. You may also be feeling anxious about the responsibility of having a baby. All this can make you feel the need to stretch and release a build-up of tension; yoga is invaluable for this, and classes that emphasise *mula bandha* (see page 170) will tone the pelvic floor .

Ask your doctor's advice at your postnatal check-up whether you are ready to start exercising again, especially if you have had a Caesarian section or a complication during the birth. If the birth was straightforward, the six-week mark is usually the point at which your body is ready, although do tell your teacher that you have given birth recently.

You may also be itching to 'get your body back', but don't be in too much of a hurry. It takes about two years before a woman's body fully returns to pre-pregnancy levels of health fitness. This is a time to get to like yourself with a tummy – not to go all out for the washboard stomach, as too much abdominal exercise too soon can have negative consequences. These muscles separate late in pregnancy to accommodate the growing baby and take time to knit together again. (If you breastfeed, though, it may help to draw the muscles back more quickly.) If your normal class emphasises core work, be extra careful not to overdo it. Exercising before the gap has closed sufficiently can

draw the muscles apart, making it worse. Your core does an important job in keeping the lower back injury-free, so again be careful that your back is not taking the strain while your abdominal muscles are weaker. Draw your pubic bone towards your navel in backbending poses such as cobra, up dog and bow so you feel your hamstrings and the base of your buttocks working. This will automatically engage your core and protect your back.

After pregnancy your ligaments will be softer than usual, due to the pregnancy hormone relaxin, making it harder for them to do their job of protecting the joints properly. Relaxin can stay in the body for weeks or months after the birth, especially if you are breastfeeding. It's important not to return to too dynamic a practice or a Yin class when your ligaments will still be very loose, as this can overextend the connective tissue and muscles that support the joints. Focus on strengthening the muscles and 'integrating' the bones back into the joints (as for 'flexible people').

Lastly, when you finally find some time to yourself to go to a yoga class, choose one that you really enjoy. Ironically, being in 'mother' mode often means we look after everyone else and forget about ourselves.

How often should I practise?

If you are looking to become stronger and/or more flexible, doing a class at least three times a week should provide measurable results – depending on the emphasis of the class (the more dynamic the class, the greater the workout). If you can make class only once a week, try to do a little of what you have learnt at home as well. There are DVDs, podcasts, apps and free YouTube content. Mornings are best, especially for a meditation practice, when you may be already calm and in a positive frame of mind. Plus, getting your practice in early on means that it's less likely to become sidelined as the day goes on.

However, there's nothing in any of the ancient teachings that says yoga has to be a 90-minute daily routine. A little every day is better than 90 minutes once a week, especially if you are looking for the more mind-based benefits such as help with stress levels.

Do I have to breathe in a special way?

In yoga we breathe through the nose, because it filters the air and allows the breath to enter the lungs fully. Good breath feeds the cells with oxygenated blood, and expels the stale carbon dioxide that can linger at the base of the lungs if our breath is shallow. It also helps keep the body alkaline (stress causes acidity – which changes the environment of the body and can weaken the immune system, making us more prone to illness).

Certainly most of us could do with learning to breathe more fully. If we are under stress, the breath becomes shallow. And if we sit for long hours hunched at our desks, the chest and ribs become compressed, and the muscles tight, limiting the space in which the lungs are able to expand. There are special breathing techniques in yoga, but trying to do them without being

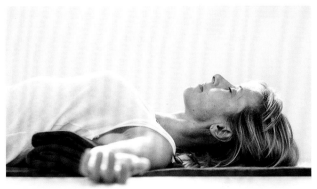

opening the chest
for better breath

able to breathe properly first is like squeezing your feet into ill-fitting shoes. It's more important to do yoga practices that open up the respiratory muscles first, such as lying on your back over a horizontally placed folded blanket to open up the chest (see below left).

Getting to know your breath by simply watching it is the first step towards learning to deepen it. Watching the breath also has a similar function to chanting in that it directs the mind to one point, taking your focus off random thoughts. Vinyasa styles, linking movement to the breath, use *ujjayi* ('victorious') breath (see page 168) as a tool for concentration. This breath gives you something to focus on; but be careful not to overdo it. It shouldn't be audible to the person next to you. *Ujjayi* has the added benefit of keeping your lower abdomen engaged, which helps protect your lower back.

Why do we salute the sun?

In ancient Indian tradition, early morning before the sun rises is seen as the most sacred and special time. Nowadays we do sun salutations (*surya namaskar*) not just in the morning classes but also at other times as a range of movements to warm up the body before going into deeper postures.

My joints click and pop when I practise. Is this good or bad?

Clicking occurs naturally, but as with anything, if it hurts, stop. Yoga anatomy specialist Paul Grilley describes two types of popping, 'friction popping' and 'fixation popping'. Friction popping is when the bones momentarily rub together, creating a vibration. There's no harm in it, but it's not good to do it habitually because it can wear the cartilage.

A 'fixation pop' happens when a joint has been immobile for some time and the lubricating fluid has been squeezed out to the sides. This creates a vacuum between the two bones, causing them to stick together. The 'pop' is the vacuum being broken. 'Fixation' makes us feel stuck or immobile in the joint (especially the fingers, toes and spine) and releasing it feels good. Grilley maintains that there is no harm in this and it is even beneficial to allow free movement of the joints.

Will I ever get my heels on the floor in downward facing dog? Does it matter?

Don't stress yourself about this, because everyone's yoga is their own and will never look exactly like other people's.

Often the reason why your heels don't reach the floor is the way you are built. People who can get their heels down easily may have a narrower angle between shin and foot and good flexibility in their back, hamstrings and calves. Bone length and depth of socket can also be a factor.

Some bodies are not made for certain poses. If you have a long body and short arms, binding your arms around your legs in a deep twist may always require a belt. Some people have a natural outward rotation to their thighs, which means sitting cross-legged or attempting lotus will be easier. They may, however, find poses such as hero pose, which rely

on internal rotation, more challenging. We are not usually a natural at both. To find out more, see the DVD *Anatomy for Yoga* by Paul Grilley.

Whichever pose you're in, learning to let go of the need to have it look like something you've seen in a book is key. I know lots of people who can get their heels down in downward dog. But are they nicer for it? Are they more enlightened? Not necessarily. Chasing ideals when you're off your mat is one thing. But taking that same attitude to your mat keeps you set on your attachments to external things – the 'look' of the pose, being 'good at yoga'. In doing this you miss the bigger point of the practice: that if all the accolades and the material trappings disappeared tomorrow, you'd still feel good about yourself.

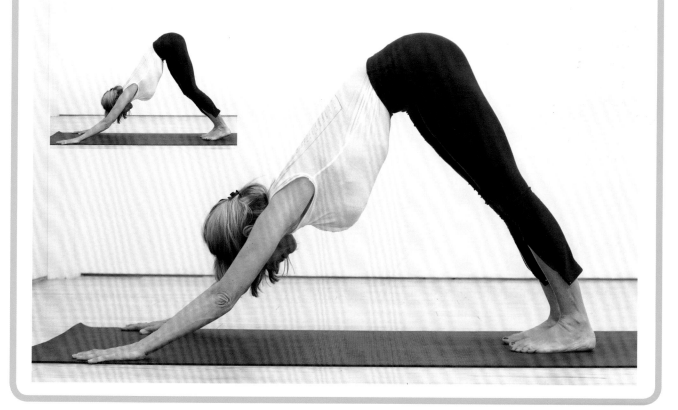

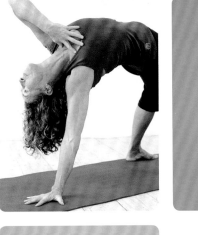

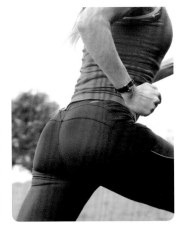
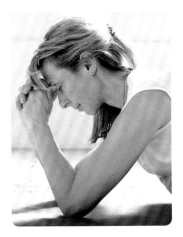
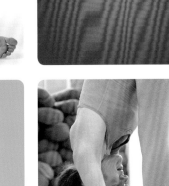
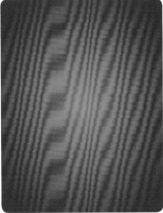
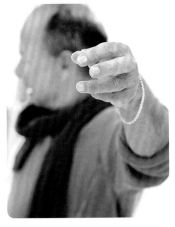

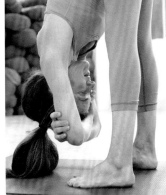

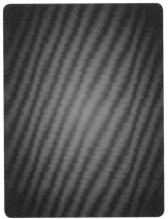
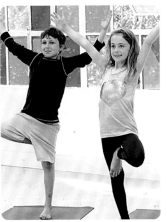

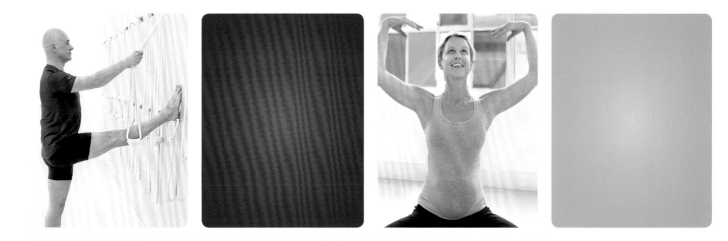

styles in focus

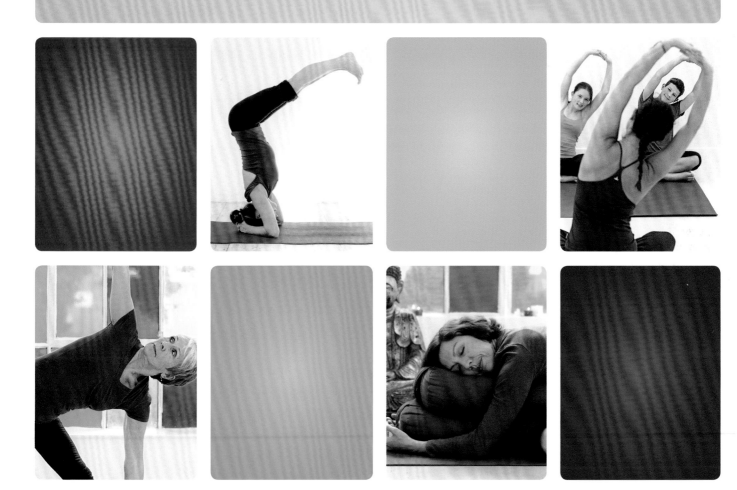

Anusara

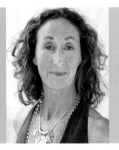

Meaning 'flowing with grace' –
Anusara is a playful, flowing,
empowering style of hatha yoga
with strong alignment principles

BY BRIDGET WOODS-KRAMER

➤ MY LIGHTBULB MOMENT

In my early twenties I set up a fashion company. It was a fickle industry and easy to feel insecure as a newcomer. A deep need for steadiness led me to an Iyengar yoga class in my local Buddhist centre. When they said, 'Stay for meditation,' I said, 'I haven't got time.' I simply wasn't ready for it.

As I became busier, the call to meditate became louder. I was giving so much to my collections, to the fitness classes I was also teaching and to my business partners, that I longed for something that gave back to me. In my mid-thirties I met my husband who took me to a Siddha Yoga meditation class. I was cynical and apprehensive – my Britishness and my conditioning said, 'This is not what you're used to.' But there was a part of me that also said, 'This feels really good.'

We all have this self-destructive voice that overrides our hearts and I didn't want to be that person any more.

I spent time in India and felt a humungous shift of energy, which they call 'shaktipat' – 'awakening'.

➤ ANUSARA IS YOGA WITH ATTITUDE

The first thing we do in Anusara is to set an intention, an offering, an attitude that infuses the practice. We chant an invocation, 'Om namah shivaya gurave,' (a Sanskrit prayer meaning 'I bow to the highest...'). This gives a sense of spiritual alignment from the outset, connecting to the greater energy that we are all part of. The poses in Anusara yoga are 'heart-oriented', so when we instruct a posture we do so from the inside out. So, for example, in triangle pose we talk about 'expanding the heart area and freeing it with the breath' rather than thinking about how it should look from the outside. This is very different from other styles that focus on aligning the body first, with the feel-good part at the end in final relaxation (savasana).

➤ FIVE 'UNIVERSAL PRINCIPLES OF ALIGNMENT'

Even though you may not notice it in class, the teacher applies these five Anusara principles sequentially in every pose in order to get the very best and most joyful expression of each one.

1. The first principle is 'attitude'. We call it 'opening to grace'; aligning with why we do the practice. This may be expressed simply by surrendering to the breath and acknowledging that we are not ultimately in control, or it may be through an inspiring or empowering theme

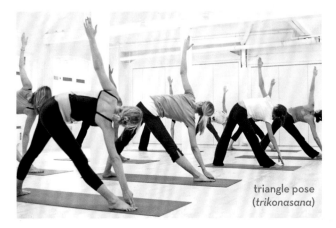

triangle pose
(trikonasana)

*We often work
together in poses.
We laugh. We might
crack a joke. The idea
is to lighten up.
We move in a way
which gives a sense
of fluidity.*

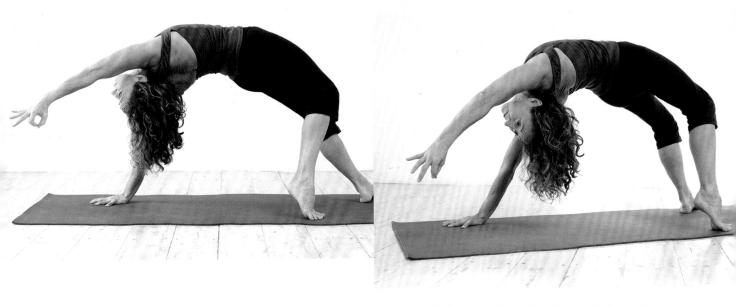

that the teacher weaves through the class.

2. The second principle is 'muscular energy' – engaging the muscles and drawing them to the bone before we stretch them, creating integration and stability in the joints. In upward facing dog, I might say, 'ground through the hands and draw up evenly on all sides of the arms into the heart region,' and you'll immediately have the feeling of integration of the bone into the shoulder joint.

3 + 4. The third and fourth principles are 'inner spiral' and 'outer spiral'. Muscles and energy don't move in straight lines, but in spirals. When we stand, most of us have our toes turned slightly out. This pushes the inner thighs forwards, creating tension around the lower back. The thighs actually have a natural inward rotation (or spiral) to them. Working with the spirals in the legs brings the pelvis and core into balance.

So, for example, in triangle pose (see page 46), we instruct you to work with the inner spiral by asking you to 'move the tops of your inner thighs back and apart'. Try it and you'll instantly feel space being created around the sacrum and back of the pelvis.

Then we ask you to scoop the tailbone under. This is applying the 'outer spiral', which is a contracting energy that starts in the waistline and draws the tailbone down. The two spirals together create *mula bandha* (see page

170) which tones the pelvic floor and draws the energy upwards through the central channel (*sushumna nadi*, see page 167).

5. The fifth principle is 'organic energy'. Unlike muscular energy, which hugs muscles in, organic energy allows us to stretch and expand out through the core lines of the body (the limbs). We can do this safely and freely if we have our focus in the right place (first principle), our muscles are engaged and joints integrated (second principle), and we have balanced action (third and fourth).

But you don't need to know any of this to enjoy Anusara. Indeed, many other styles are now using its terminology because they have seen that the universal principles of alignment really work.

I have practised Anusara for years because I've seen it biomechanically align people's bodies and allow an optimal flow of energy.

Through this method, its founder John Friend has healed countless injuries (back injuries, such as disc problems and sciatic pain, shoulder injuries, knee injuries, tennis elbow, carpal tunnel problems and so on) because it aligns the bones correctly, it places engagement of muscles before extension, and looks for balanced action in the muscles, bones as well as energy body.

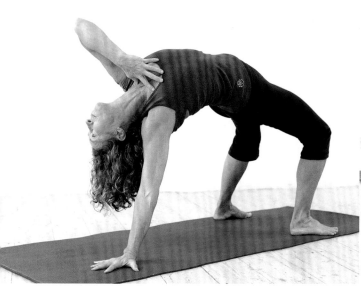

➤ WE DON'T TAKE OURSELVES TOO SERIOUSLY

Anusara is a playful celebration of the spirit. An Anusara teacher is committed to empowering students and building their self-esteem, while inspiring light-heartedness, play and joyful creativity within the yoga practice. We often work together in poses. We laugh. We might crack a joke. The idea is to lighten up. We move in a way which gives people a sense of fluidity, so classes tend to follow a flowing vinyasa style. That's not to say you always have to feel playful. Anusara is about honouring how you feel. You might come to class feeling angry because you've lost your job, or heartbroken over a relationship or sad for any number of reasons. Just being with your emotions and letting them move through you as you breathe and flow through your postures can help you feel lighter.

➤ OPENING THE HEART AND THE HIPS

If you have experienced physical trauma, the body will start to tighten around an injury. Emotional traumas are the same. If you've been hurt or are afraid, it might reflect in your posture, in a rounding of the shoulders to protect the heart. We store a lot in our hips too. It's said that childhood traumas reside there. That's not to say that everyone with tight hips is carrying emotional baggage. But often when we do hip openers or heart openers (such as backbends) we may well feel an emotional release. We don't have to analyse why.

Western lifestyle factors – especially computers and chairs – have a lot to answer for when it comes to tightness in the hips and heart region. Much of what we do these days is 'forward facing'. Hunching over our desks and computers tightens up the front of the body, and sitting on chairs tightens our hip flexor muscles. It takes the natural curve out of our lower back and causes sluggish circulation in the lower body. In Anusara yoga, you'll find plenty of heart- and hip-openers.

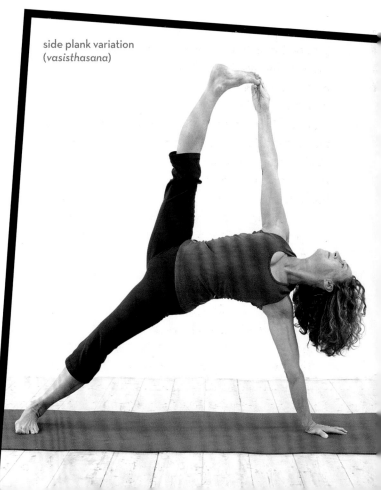

side plank variation
(vasisthasana)

⏰ if you only have ten minutes

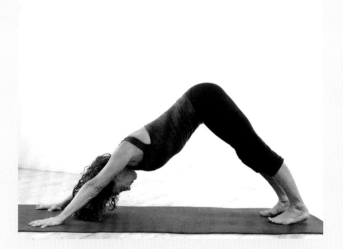

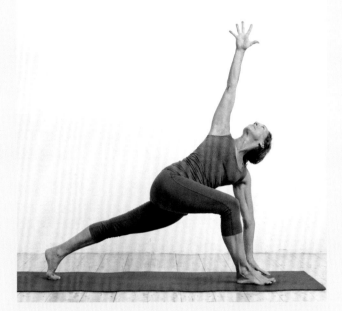

1. DOWNWARD FACING DOG

From all fours, arms straight, draw the shoulder blades down the back, tuck the toes under, lift knees and extend back into downward facing dog. With the knees slightly bent, lift your sitbones and stretch the hips back, lengthening through the sides of the torso and spine. Then begin to straighten the legs and root down from the pelvis without losing the extension through the spine. Breathe here for a while.

2. TWISTING LUNGE

From downward facing dog, step the right foot forwards into lunge, lengthen the spine and twist to the right, raising the right arm to the sky, shoulder blades curling into the back of your heart as you breathe and open up the lungs. Let go of any tension in the mind. Come back to downward facing dog and repeat on the other side.

3. TWISTING LUNGE WITH THIGH STRETCH

From downward facing dog, stretch one leg up and back to open up the hips, then step it forward into a low lunge, placing the back knee on the floor. Hold the foot of the back leg and draw it into the buttock to stretch the thigh. Repeat on the other side.

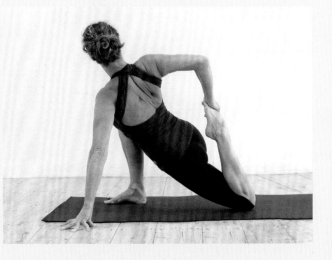

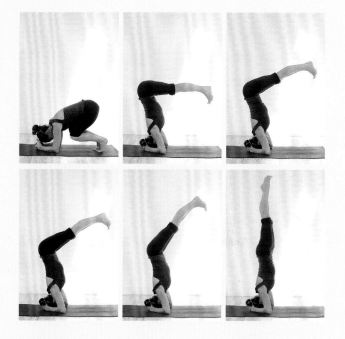

4. PIGEON

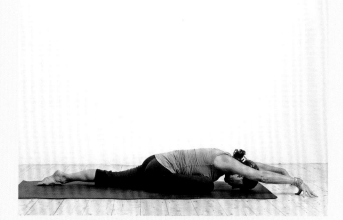

From downward facing dog, inhale, raise the right leg, bend the right knee and bring it to the floor behind your right wrist. Take the right foot across the mat towards your left hand, with pelvis and hips square to the front of the mat. Scoop the tailbone down, lengthen through the spine, lift the heart. Extend through the back leg and support the right buttock with a cushion if you find yourself collapsing over to the right. Bow forwards, lengthen through the spine, forehead to the floor. Press the fingertips down, lift the elbows and armpits away from the floor. Melt the heart towards the floor.

Stay here for five breaths. Repeat on the other side. If you have knee issues, take eye of the needle pose (see page 155).

5. HEADSTAND

If I've had a busy day or have been travelling, headstand brings my energy right back in. Your mind can't go anywhere otherwise you will fall. By rooting down through the arms, lifting the shoulders up away from the floor and grounding through the upper palate and crown of your head, the spine naturally lengthens. Take headstand for 20 breaths if you have learnt this pose from a teacher. If it is not yet in your practice, take downward facing dog with the crown of your head resting on a block. Both are powerful grounding and centring poses.

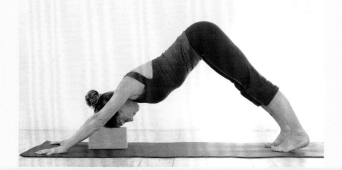

Ashtanga

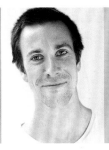

A dynamic and challenging sequence that follows a set pattern, synchronises breath with movement and builds internal heat to detoxify the body

BY JOEY MILES

➤ MY LIGHTBULB MOMENT

I was 16 in the late 1990s and working part-time in a juggling shop; there was one guy who was so much better at juggling than everyone else. When I asked my boss why, he said, 'He doesn't drink alcohol and he does yoga.' I hadn't considered that yoga could work in a deeply practical way. Maybe it could not only improve my juggling but transform my ability to concentrate too and generally make me feel really good. So I got a book and copied the shapes every morning for about 30 minutes. I had the idea of replacing a negative habit (smoking) with a positive one (yoga), so I never skipped my morning postures. My whole body was stiff, but the way it released amazed me. It wasn't just a physical transformation; my mental health seemed to improve a hundred-fold.

At university in London I found an Ashtanga class. My teacher encouraged me to try 'Mysore style', where students work through postures in the Ashtanga primary series at their own pace. At my first class I copied those around me for a while and then did my own thing. The teacher scolded me for not following the set sequence. She showed me up to *marichyasana* D (see below left) – a seated twist about halfway into the sequence – and told me to stop there. As I was leaving she said, 'Hey, do not come back unless you learn the sequence... and you'd better come back!'

I found the diagram of the primary series which for so long I'd gone through randomly, skipping the harder poses, and every day I went up to *marichyasana* D until I could do it and was ready to add the next pose. Now I was on the Ashtanga path, learning the traditional method of adding one pose at a time, only going as far through the primary series as I could go with integrity.

➤ IT'S CHALLENGING, FAST-MOVING MEDITATION IN MOTION

Ashtanga is a dynamic class that follows a set pattern. The aim of the primary series (or *yoga chikitsa* – there are more advanced series too) is to purify the body and mind and realign the musculoskeletal system. It begins with sun salutations, which are essentially a moving prayer – or a movement meditation. They lead into a set of standing postures, such as triangle and warrior. The seated poses that follow are primarily forward bends, often done with modifications, because most of us have stiff feet, ankles, knees and hips. The poses aren't held for long (five breaths) but there are lots of them. The emphasis is always on the link between breath (*ujjayi*,

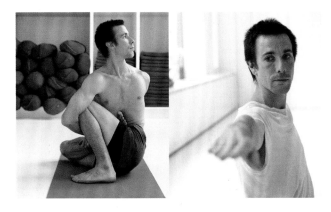

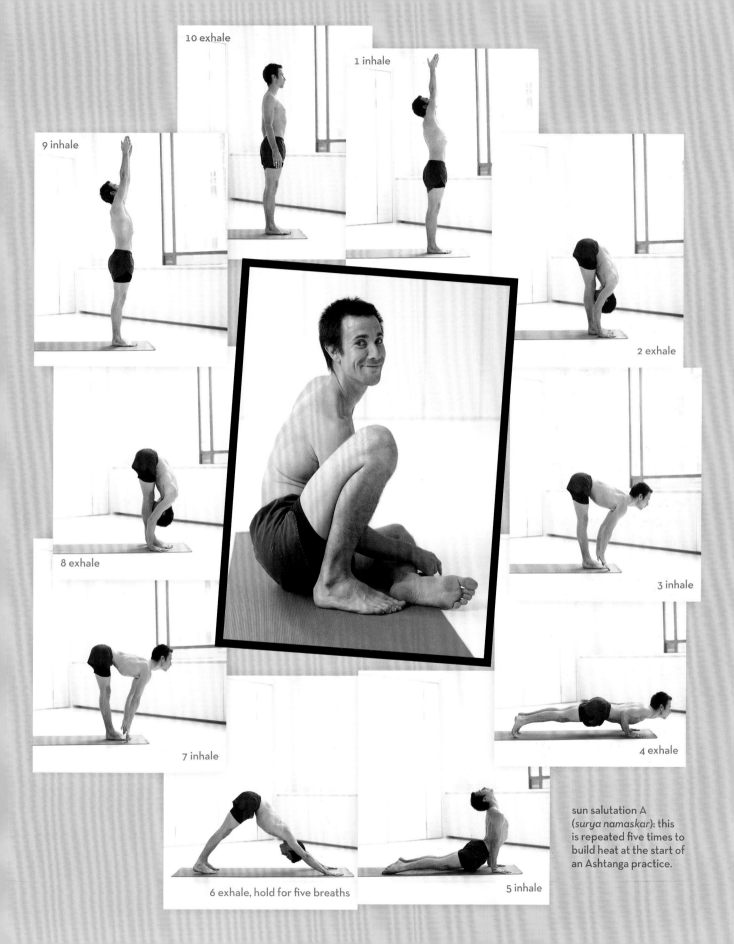

10 exhale

1 inhale

9 inhale

2 exhale

8 exhale

3 inhale

7 inhale

4 exhale

6 exhale, hold for five breaths

5 inhale

sun salutation A
(*surya namaskar*): this
is repeated five times to
build heat at the start of
an Ashtanga practice.

dropping back into
upward facing bow

jumping through
from downward
facing dog to sitting

see page 168) and movement. When done well, it's like a fluid dance.

It is a physical and mental challenge for anyone; but by following the sequence you quickly see yourself change and progress. Because the sequence sticks in your memory, it's quite easy to practise at home because you know what you are supposed to be doing.

In 'Mysore style' there are lots of hands-on adjustments and fewer verbal instructions, so the room is quiet and focused. I encourage people to use props if needed (this is frowned upon and seen as not traditional by some). Being a pragmatist, I can't see the sense in making it harder than it needs to be.

There is a widely held misconception about Ashtanga, that there's one set sequence that won't be changed for anyone. But through the 'Mysore style' self-practice method, a teacher gives each student only what is within their capacity. So, by being told to stop at an appropriate point, we can learn that less is more, and it needn't be such a struggle.

> ASHTANGA MEANS 'EIGHT LIMBS'

The Ashtanga lineage is currently upheld by my teacher in Mysore, Sharath Jois, at the Sri K Pattabhi Jois Ashtanga Yoga Institute, named after his late grandfather, the style's founder. Anyone can apply to study there and I highly recommend it. Most students go to practise the *asanas*, but there are also Sanskrit chanting classes. This helps put the practice into its wider context, so we learn it's not about body perfection but about becoming a better person. The physical practice acts as a mirror, reflecting how we're doing as a person. When I feel I'm in a big hurry on the

mat, I know I also need to slow down in my whole life.

Ashtanga means eight limbs, a term that comes from Patanjali's *Yoga Sutras*, describing the eight elements of yoga. The implication of this (to me) is that there are many ways to get to the state of yoga, and that they all interlink. Pattabhi Jois ('Guruji') always said that for us the main route is *asana* – the third of the eight limbs. 'Practise and all is coming,' was his answer to most people's questions and doubts. He knew that with commitment and practice we discover that the postures are fuelled by breath (*pranayama*, the fourth limb) and that the gateways to the senses – the eyes, ears, nose, mouth and skin – relax and turn inwards (*pratyahara*, the fifth limb). Without concentration (*dharana*, the sixth limb) you get nowhere and the practice simply won't flow without meditation (*dhyana*, the seventh limb). And if we didn't keep getting little tastes of *samadhi* (ecstasy, the eighth limb), I'm not sure if the motivation would stay as strong – but it certainly does for me!

That leaves the first two limbs – *yama* (restraint) and *niyama* (observance). They give us deeply practical guidance on how to live; how to relate to ourselves, to others and to the world. It's no use perfecting *asanas* and ignoring the problems around us. But by starting with ourselves, we can make the world a nicer place – practising kindness, honesty and so on.

➤ 'EVERYONE CAN DO THIS PRACTICE EXCEPT LAZY PEOPLE!'

That's what my teacher Sharath said. And it's true. The type of people who take to Ashtanga instantly love the fire element; they like adrenaline and challenge. Addictive personality types love it, but need to be careful. When you practise for two hours a day, six days a week, it can take over your life. This is why we take a day off from practice twice a month, during the full and new moons.

Yoga taking over your life a little isn't so bad, but becoming too attached to anything turns it into a crutch. So we aim to cultivate detachment. I remember one lady in Mysore becoming very agitated at not having done her practice for a few days. She asked Guruji what could be done if travelling kept you off the mat for two or three days. He just laughed and said, 'Why not read a book?'

Ashtanga is a strong practice but it's not just for the physically fit. Over the past ten years I have seen people receive such benefit from the practice; people with cancer, HIV and AIDS; some coming to the mat after paralysing spinal injury, addiction, divorce or mental breakdown.

➤ WHY COUNTING COUNTS

I have a love for the tradition and the bare bones of the practice, the simplicity of the breath and the counting in Sanskrit. In Mysore, where the classes are now so big, the week begins and ends with a 'counted' class. Here, the teacher calls the breath movement (*vinyasa*) number and everyone does their best to stay in time. Staying aware of the count is like following sheet music or being in a band; you have to be part of the collective movement. It is a powerful tool for progressing in Ashtanga as it requires mind control to stop you zoning out and daydreaming.

➤ BUT IT SHOULDN'T BECOME YOGA-BY-NUMBERS

When I find myself and my students becoming mechanical (a big trap in yoga and life), I do my best to be playful, to speed it up or slow it right down, turn out the lights or use blindfolds or music. Yoga is a dense, complex subject, but the paradox is that when we take it, or ourselves, too seriously we can't even get close. So stop trying to look cool doing yoga, wear bad shorts and tuck your vest into your pants! Don't be in a hurry, and practise a little bit every single day – for ever.

if you only have ten minutes

SUN SALUTATIONS

Remind yourself why it is you do yoga (aim for the highest!) and then set an intention. Make it really simple: for example, 'Can I practise today with gentleness and be kind to myself?' Get a copy of the Ashtanga primary series from a book or download it from the internet. Copy the poses in order. Do sun salutation A (shown on page 53) and sun salutation B three times, and keep going with the sequence for as long as you have time, taking only three breaths in each pose. Sit down and listen to the even, steady *ujjayi* breath sound. Then let it all go as you lie down and rest for a few minutes. It might feel like paying a hurried visit to a friend. You don't really stay long enough, but it's good to drop in all the same.

hatha

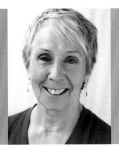

A general yoga class in which the emphasis reflects the teacher's influences and interests

BY LOUISE GRIME

➤ MY LIGHTBULB MOMENT

I was 27 and in a very stressful job managing restaurants. I drank and smoked a little too much and always seemed to be nursing a cough. I couldn't touch my knees, let alone my toes. When a friend took me to my first class in an adult education centre with a local Iyengar yoga teacher, something about it struck a chord. I didn't realise just how badly I'd needed it. It got rid of a lot of stress. Pretty quickly the cigarettes and alcohol dropped away. I went back to college, which led to a career in theatre and then television. Being freelance meant that I could take months off between jobs and in 1989 I went to the Sivananda Ashram in Kerala, India, to do their teacher training, initially more out of a desire to learn than to teach. It was the start of my lifelong journey of becoming a happier, healthier, more aware person – of finding my self. Without yoga I wouldn't have challenged myself so much. It encourages you to explore the boundaries of what you can do both on and off the mat.

➤ HATHA IS ALL PHYSICAL YOGA

If you see hatha yoga advertised on a class schedule (it may simply be called yoga), the class can vary depending on where you go and who the teacher is. When we talk about hatha yoga we mean the physical path; but it is only one way to reach the ultimate goal of yoga – the peaceful feeling of connectedness with the universe. In India, people follow other paths that lead to the same end state, such as *karma* yoga (helping

others), *bhakti* yoga (devotional practices such as chanting) or *jnana* yoga (studying the self and the yogic texts). Different paths suit different personalities. But in the West we tend to be drawn to the physical practice of yoga because we are familiar with exercise as a way of improving wellbeing. Hatha yoga is part of a path known as *raja* (royal) yoga, which combines postures, *pranayama* (breathing), meditation and living the yoga philosophy.

In general, a hatha session might begin seated or lying on the mat and tuning into your breath, followed by gentle stretches. A warm-up practice including sun salutations is followed by standing poses, such as triangle (see right) and warrior, with twists, standing balances, forward bending and backbending all thrown into the mix, and the session ends with final relaxation. This is the time when all the benefits of the practice are able to take effect. A morning practice will normally be energising for the day ahead, an evening practice calming in preparation for sleep. I bring in breathing exercises and positive thought as well as elements of yoga philosophy (especially the eight limbs, see page 18) since yoga is much more than what you do on the mat.

➤ HATHA IS ABOUT BALANCE

Hatha is a good 'way in' to yoga for Westerners. It's about balancing the body – left and right, front and back ('*ha*' means sun and '*tha*' means moon in Sanskrit), but we are also balancing the emotions and the mind.

you start to see the world from different perspectives – quite literally, when you are looking up in triangle pose, or are upside down in headstand

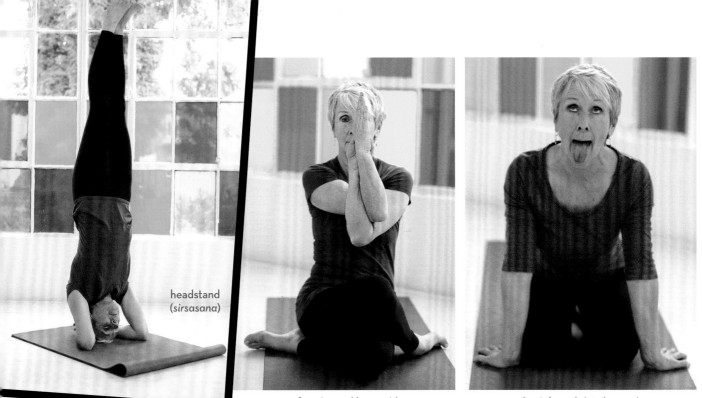

headstand
(*sirsasana*)

cow face (*gomukhasana*) legs
with eagle (*garudasana*) arms

lion's breath (*simhasana*)

The reason why we do these physical practices is so that we reach higher levels of understanding of ourselves and can sit comfortably in meditation. If your body is very tense or unbalanced how can you sit quietly? But even if you don't do specific meditation practice, hatha yoga reduces stress and brings about a more balanced approach to every aspect of your life.

➤ YOGA SHOULD MAKE YOU FEEL GOOD

Some schools of hatha have a specific brand name coined by the teacher responsible for a particular emphasis, such as Ashtanga vinyasa, Iyengar yoga, Shadow yoga or Sivananda. They are very different, yet all come under the umbrella of hatha and usually include the yogic philosophical principles. Different styles might work for different stages in your life. I used to love Ashtanga and did the Mysore self-practice class six days a week. But when I reached the age of 50 and began teaching full time, it prompted me to think a little more about what my body needed and to adapt what I was doing into a home practice that felt good for me. Doing yoga should make you feel happy and comfortable in your body. It doesn't matter whether

or not you can get yourself into some tricky posture. For me, *asana* practice is about keeping my body comfortable to live in so I can conduct my life in a contented, aware manner and fulfil everything I want to do.

➤ IT'S A JOURNEY THAT STARTS WITH THE BODY

On a basic level, yoga lets you get to know your body. You might begin to realise that you favour one leg more than the other or that when you are standing you stick one hip out. Knowing ourselves physically means we are better able to take our place in the world comfortably. If you are more comfortable in yourself, you start to enquire what's going on inside. Many of us avoid looking inwards – especially when we lack confidence or feel negatively about ourselves. But knowing yourself is an important part of yoga. It's surprising what you discover when you sit quietly and watch the breath. You might find yourself thinking, 'Hang on a minute, why am I projecting all these emotions – anger, disappointment, envy – on to other people, when the only way to find contentment is within myself?' Once you start to spend a little time every day sitting and knowing yourself, you're an easier person to get on with. Ultimately it's about taking responsibility for yourself.

➤ STEADY BREATH, STEADY MIND

On the mat we learn how focusing on the breath quietens the mind. Because yoga filters into your way of thinking off the mat, you will find yourself using it as a tool in everyday life too. Watching the breath helps you to think more clearly and make more measured decisions. In a road-rage situation, for example, you might find yourself quite naturally coming back to the breath. Instead of cutting up the car in front, you might put on some uplifting music and start singing or chanting. I give my students facial yoga exercises to do in the car. Lion's breath (a strong exhale with mouth and eyes wide and tongue stretched out fully) is good if you hold tension in the jaw (it also helps alleviate bad breath and makes your diction clearer). If you are in a traffic jam going nowhere, you can make a choice. You can be really fed up or you can do breathing exercises and change your outlook on the situation. Yoga teaches us the art of turning negative experiences and thoughts into positive ones, to step back and not always to react – to be more mindful generally.

➤ YOGA IS YOU – BUT BETTER

The yoga scriptures talk about 'liberation' and connecting with your 'higher self' but it's not something you need to know to enjoy yoga. As Pattabhi Jois, the founder of Ashtanga vinyasa, said: 'Practise and all is coming.' As you start to practise regularly, your body starts to open up. You breathe more fully and you start to become more used to seeing the world from different perspectives (quite literally, when you are looking up in triangle pose, or are upside down in headstand). You also start to know yourself better. Time and again I have seen students becoming more confident, standing taller, their chests opening, having energy and sparkling eyes – becoming more their true selves. Yoga allows you to drop your armour in class. And once you have been practising for some time, you may find that you don't need that armour in the outside world either.

if you only have ten minutes

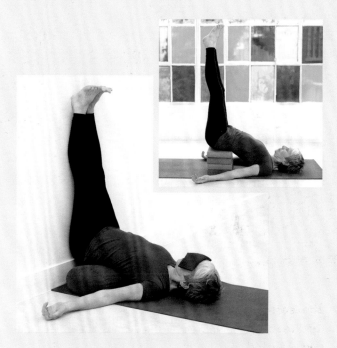

LEGS-UP-THE-WALL (*viparita karani*)

The pose I always come back to is *viparita karani* (legs-up-the-wall). I love this pose because I tend to close my chest and lying like this for ten minutes helps me breathe and quietens me. Its benefits are many and varied – among them are relieving anxiety, helping with digestive problems and high and low blood pressure, and so it goes on. It can help relieve tired legs if you've been on your feet all day, and also help you sleep.

To do it, lie with your legs up the wall and a bolster under your buttocks. Or for a more challenging version, place three or four stacked blocks under your sacrum (the flat bone at the base of your spine). Legs can be unsupported in the air or resting against the wall. Place your hands wherever is comfortable alongside the body. Watch the breath.

Avoid this pose if you have glaucoma, have had eye surgery or have serious back or neck problems. If you have your period and prefer not to practise inversions, you may like to remove the bolster or blocks.

Iyengar yoga

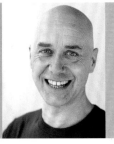

A safe, progressive and vigorous method of *asana* (postures) and *pranayama*

BY ALARIC NEWCOMBE

➤ MY LIGHTBULB MOMENT

In 1983 I had just finished my first degree and was about to travel to Egypt to teach English and I wanted an exercise manual to take with me. The book that caught my eye was *Light on Yoga* by BKS Iyengar. I noticed that the practice sequences were spread over six years, and when I saw how advanced the postures became I thought, 'Wow! This will keep me going for the rest of my life.' I started the standing sequences and was astonished at how my mood and experience of myself were transformed. I quickly realised that it was as much an exercise for mind as for body. I was hooked.

BKS Iyengar, his son and a daughter have been exploring and expanding their teaching for decades. His is a varied and versatile system that makes life-long learning possible. This is what I was looking for. I practised every day for five years from *Light on Yoga* before returning to the UK to take classes and later to train as a teacher.

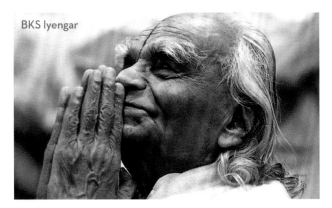

BKS Iyengar

➤ WE TAKE TIME TO EXPLORE EACH POSTURE

A hallmark of Iyengar yoga is respect for the postures (*asana*) – building them up safely and exploring them internally and externally. Iyengar yoga teachers spend time showing you how to set up postures properly, first by demonstration and giving key points verbally. Then the students do it for themselves and the teacher repeats the instructions and physically adjusts if necessary in order to make the posture anatomically correct and create coherence within the body/mind of the student.

➤ ALWAYS START WITH AN IYENGAR YOGA BEGINNERS' CLASS, EVEN IF YOU HAVE DONE OTHER YOGA BEFORE

Sometimes people who come to class have not learned *asana* mindfully. They sometimes feel frustrated by their own practice, asking, 'Why am I unable to stay in shoulder stand or headstand for ten minutes?' or they are puzzled as to why they have repeated injury or can't sit even for a short *pranayama* practice. They may well have missed basic principles. I recommend a beginners' class, where you can learn to build up the *asana* in the correct way – and stay in them longer. The inner body, the organs, the nerves and the mind all become strengthened and replenished through Iyengar's method. The purpose of doing the *asana* well is for all the layers of our being to be healed so that the spiritual qualities within naturally and spontaneously become

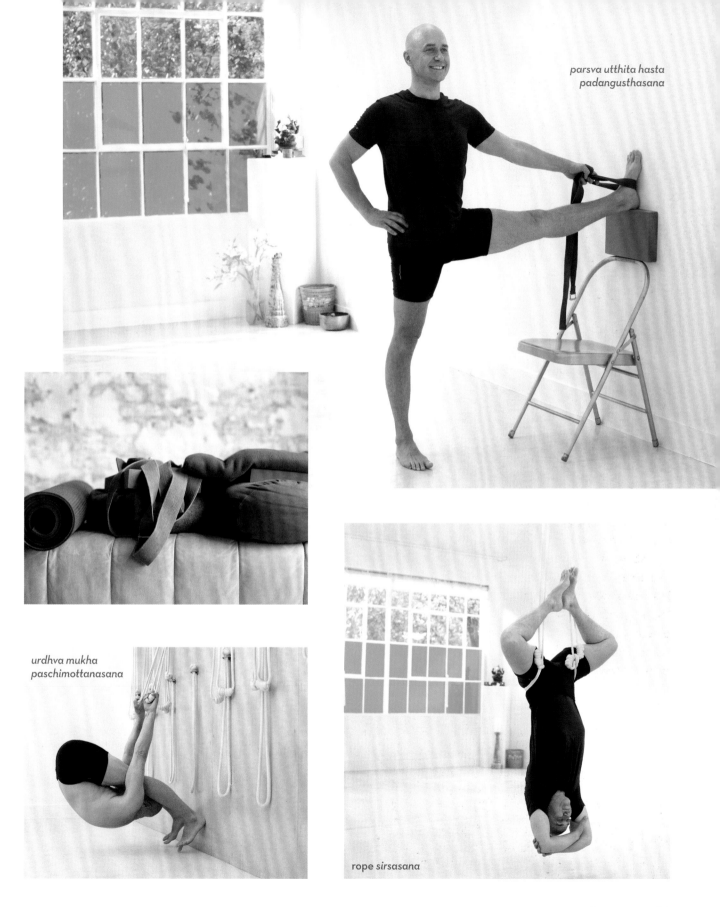

*parsva utthita hasta
padangusthasana*

*urdhva mukha
paschimottanasana*

rope sirsasana

manifest. This isn't possible if we are mentally distracted and physically depleted by energetic imbalances in the body and mind.

➤ WARMING UP WITH SHOULDER AND CHEST STRETCHES

Beginners start by taking the arms out wide and overhead. For Westerners this is often difficult because we spend a lot of time sitting at desks with our shoulders slumped forwards and chest compressed. Some sports can also cause stiffness in this area. These stretches improve breathing by extending the intercostal muscles. If you can get used to being big in the heart and holding the chest open, the way you approach other people – and life – will improve.

➤ STRONG LEGS, STRONG SPINE, STRONG MIND

The beginner is often weak and loose, or strong but stiff. We give a lot of standing poses to develop stability in the body as well as mobility in the hips and legs. (Iyengar often teaches the standing postures wide – see below – so there is stretching of the legs, pelvis and spine.) Strong legs are important for the nervous system because the spine – which contains much of it – depends on the legs for stability. Because the brain sits on the spine, and the spine depends on the legs, the meditative qualities of yoga start with the feet and legs.

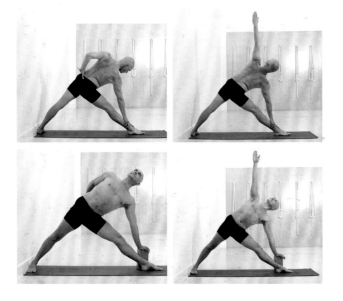

➤ POSTURES ARE FOR EVERYONE, NOT JUST FLEXIBLE PEOPLE

There's a picture from the early 1960s of BKS Iyengar helping his student, the violinist Yehudi Menuhin, with *setu bandha sarvangasana* (bridge posture). Menuhin isn't able to get his feet to the floor with his chest open, so Iyengar supports his hips with his hand. When Iyengar started teaching larger classes he wasn't able to hold everyone, so to make the *asana* accessible to them, and to enable them to find space and extension, he would use the occasional prop. He introduced the idea of doing a shoulder stand on several folded blankets because he wanted people to experience the opening in the chest and space in the lungs more fully. If the lungs lift, the body and brain are energised and soothed, not strained. The posture can then be restorative.

The props he used were whatever was around. Many classes were taught in gymnasia and school halls, so the obvious things were gym mats and wall ropes; or a bolster might be used – the sort that can be found in Indian homes.

I sometimes call props 'fillips' because they should stimulate you into the posture. In some methods, if someone can't do a posture, they might skip it, or do it in a way that causes injury. An Iyengar yoga teacher will show you a way to do the *asana* so that you may and can benefit from the entire range of movements.

➤ WHY WE STAY IN POSTURES LONGER

Iyengar found that staying longer in *asana* – which is sometimes easier with a prop – works the body more thoroughly, making the blood flow through the many layers of muscle as well as within the organs. The student can then experience relaxation as well as activation throughout the body.

People often say that Iyengar yoga practitioners are perfectionist about doing postures well – and, yes, we try to be. The reason is that the body is considered a temple and the *asana* the prayers. When we stay in a posture longer and treat it as a meditative object, it takes on a spiritual form, becoming like a *ruupa* (a term denoting beauty applied to statues of deities).

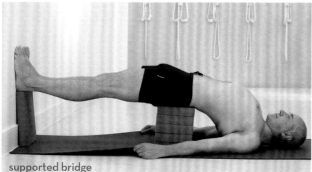

supported bridge
(*setu bandha sarvangasana*)

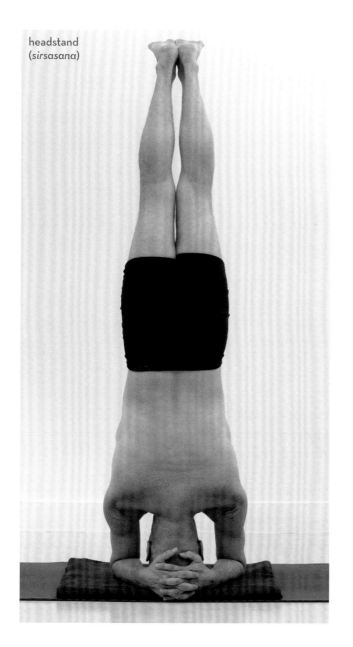

headstand
(*sirsasana*)

➤ YOGA HELPS THE BODY HEAL ITSELF

As a young man, Iyengar suffered from malaria, typhoid and tuberculosis – and used yoga to bring himself to full health. He has a particular interest in medical yoga classes, where students come with all manner of conditions such as severe arthritis, heart disease, depression and so on. He enjoys the challenge presented to him when medical cases tell him, 'There's nothing anyone can do for me.' Iyengar gives *asana* as a way of supporting the body's capacity to heal itself – by improving the blood flow and boosting the immune system, for example. For him the *asana* are like X-rays, allowing him to see what's going on inside the body. Because this type of 'seeing' requires great experience and understanding, he has stipulated that only teachers who have passed assessments beyond their initial teaching qualification are able to address serious medical conditions using his name.

shoulder stand on folded blankets
(*salamba sarvangasana*)

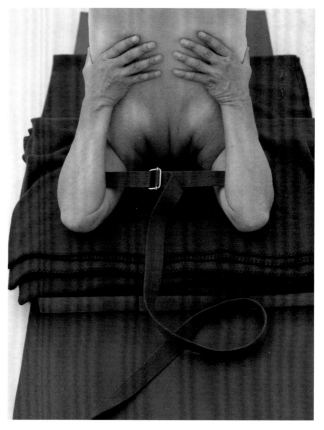

⏱ *if you only have ten minutes*

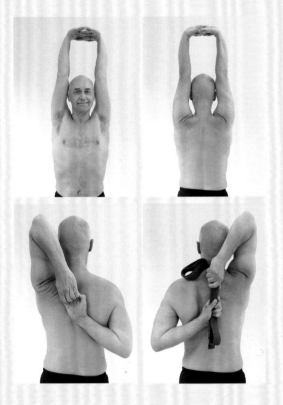

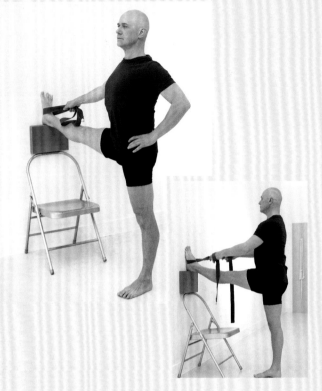

STANDING SHOULDER STRETCHES

These are a good way to start any practice. Linking the hands, turn the palms away, stretch your fingers and strongly extend the arms straight up. Check in a mirror that they are not bent. Make sure your trapezius muscles (where shoulders meet the neck) move down away from your neck. Lower the arms and change the interlace of the fingers and repeat several times.

Next bend one arm behind your back, raise the other behind your head and hold hands or fingers. Keep your shoulders level and your shoulder blades flat into your back. You may need to hold a belt between the hands to achieve the goal, which is level shoulders and flat shoulder blades. Do both sides.

LEG RAISES

During sleep, the spinal discs become more filled with fluid, a frequent cause of morning back pain. Leg raises extend the legs and activate the spine and sciatic nerve, undoing compression.

— **leg raise to the side:** With the right side of your body leg-distance from the wall, turn the right leg out to 90 degrees, raise it and place it on a chair, windowsill, kitchen worktop or other support. Loop a belt around your foot and pull on the belt so your shoulder blades and spine press into the back to open the chest. Keeping your hips level and square to the room is the real challenge. Keep your standing foot parallel to the wall and both knees firm. Change legs.

— **leg raise facing the wall:** Stand leg-distance from the wall. Raise your left leg and place your heel on the support. Keep your standing foot at a right angle to the wall, both knees firm. Hold the belt with both hands. Change legs.

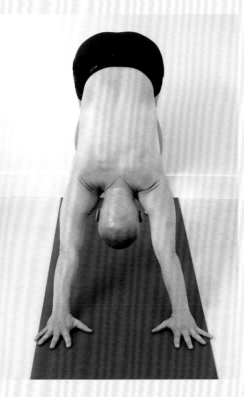

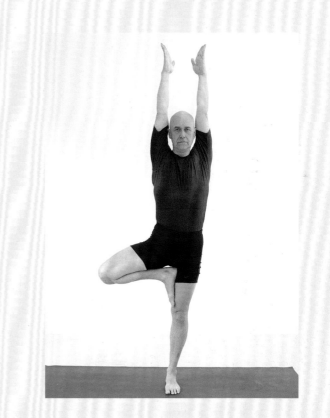

DOG POSE

The goal of this *asana* is to lengthen the whole of the trunk and spine by strongly lifting the hips up and back. Straighten and lift the arms and press the legs back as much as you can. Move the upper back towards your thighs. Don't worry if your head touches the floor, you can use a blanket for support.

TREE POSTURE

Do this with completely straight arms and lift the whole body up while gripping your outer hips. Make sure the hips stay square to the room. The bent-leg knee moves back (not your pelvis).

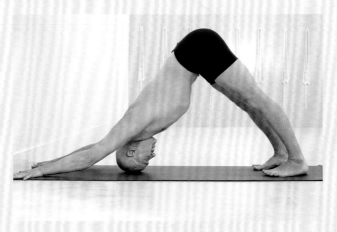

Hopefully this sequence will take eight minutes. Use the last two minutes to organise attendance at an Iyengar yoga class and to study *Yoga the Iyengar Way* by Silva, Mira and Shyam Mehta, one of the best home-practice books available.

yoga *for kids to teens*

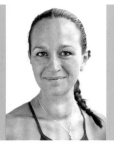

Yoga helps children handle the stresses of a competitive and technology-centric age as well as the physical and emotional pressures of growing up. It can improve coordination, strength, posture, concentration, confidence and memory (and it's fun!)

BY SUSANNAH HOFFMAN

➤ MY LIGHTBULB MOMENT

Yoga and meditation have always been part of me – I was born to the sound of my mother chanting. My parents were interested in Eastern philosophies and taught me and my siblings to listen to our inner guidance and to understand that there was always a bigger picture. When I was growing up I felt like two halves, at odds with my friends and surroundings and full of questions about the universe. I became a professional dancer but at 23 gave up dance to focus only on yoga and meditation, and that was when the two halves of me – the physical and the spiritual – began to integrate. Even now, if I don't practise for a few days, I start to feel a little disconnected.

My own experience has made me very aware of how too many children – and also adults – lack a sense of connection. I saw it clearly in my early twenties, when I taught on a series of summer dance and drama workshops for kids. I was shocked to find that at age five they already doubted their abilities. They would rather not try something than get it wrong. I introduced

simple yoga postures such as hissing cobra, cat and tree – poses that every child could do without being competitive. I encouraged them not only to try but also to enjoy trying and to experience a feeling of achievement whatever their ability. They loved it and many of them carried on doing yoga with me into their teens, some even wanting to become yoga teachers.

➤ AGES TWO TO THREE AND A HALF:
inspired by nature

For very little ones yoga is a fast-moving class, centred on postures drawn from the natural world, such as cat, cow, lion, cobra, dog, butterfly and tree. It helps them with both gross and fine motor skills and encourages imagination. Toddlers are in no way expected to sit still and meditate, but making animal sounds such as 'moo' lengthens the breath and helps calm the mind. Standing on one leg pretending to be a tree brings balance and focus. Children are very receptive to sound, so it's easy to introduce chanting such as '*Om*' at the beginning of the class, ending with '*Om shanti*' ('peace').

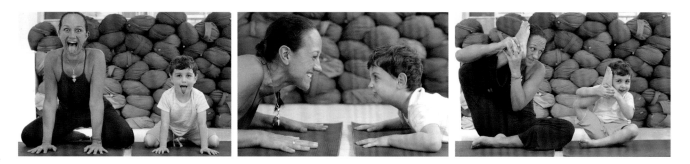

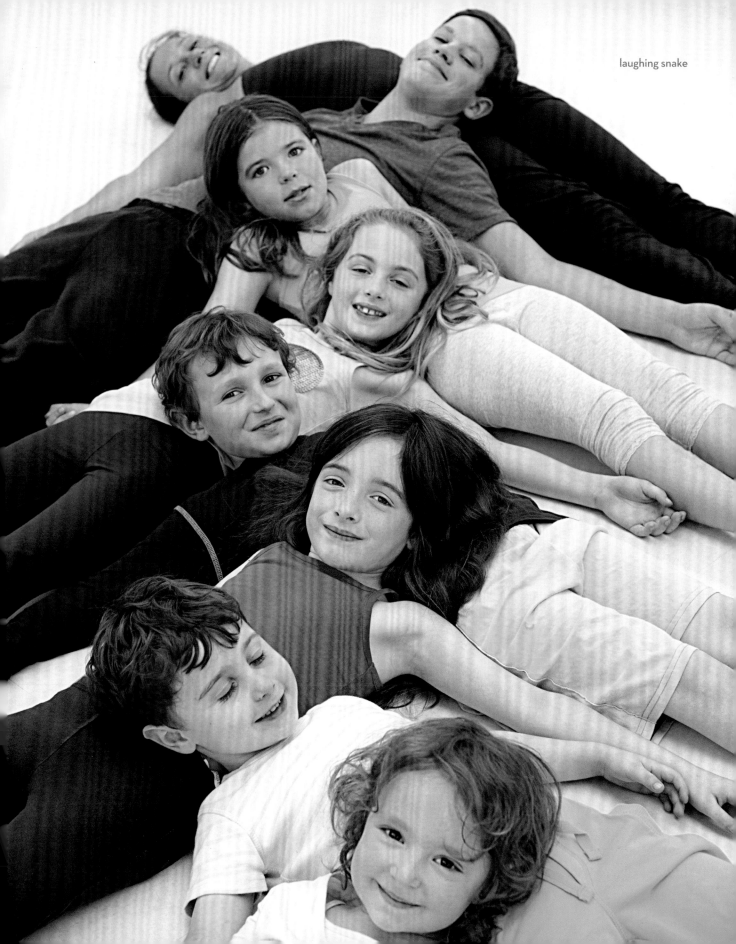

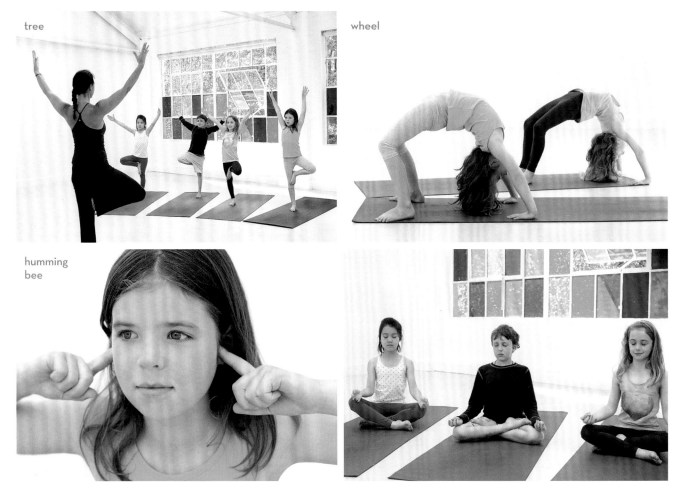

tree

wheel

humming
bee

➤ AGES FOUR TO SIX: sound, silence, magic and wonder

Here, children are introduced to relaxation by making themselves melt like ice cream or be as floppy as spaghetti. We work with sound (long exhalations encourage relaxation) as well as with silence, which is so rare in their lives. Moving with no sound at all in yoga creates a magical atmosphere and teaches them to be comfortable with silence. At this age, they have a strong sense of magic and awe. I encourage them to have confidence in themselves and their ideas. They are still very flexible, so we try to maintain it with exercises such as 'magic pot' (see page 71).

➤ AGES SEVEN TO NINE: getting to know their breath

Children's lungs do not fully develop until around age eight. Because a full breath is linked to concentration,

it's physically impossible for a child to sit still for any length of time before this age. Now we introduce simple breathing techniques such as *brahmari* (humming bee breath, page 71) which calms the mind and helps concentration. They learn to improve the length of their exhale week by week without becoming competitive. Yoga is a powerful way to show children that everyone progresses at their own speed. I remind them that some will find tree pose easier, while others are able to do a really strong warrior – and that it doesn't matter.

Guided relaxation and visualisations help with the language of feelings and listening to their inner guidance. They are asked to hold up an imaginary crystal to the sun, to give it the first colour that comes into their mind and then to visualise that colour shining down on them. If they choose to tell me how it makes them feel, they say things like 'happy', 'peaceful', 'brave'.

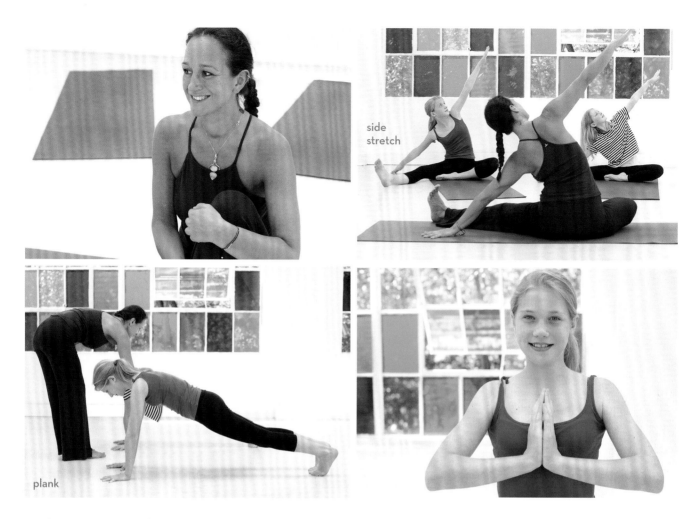

side stretch

plank

It's also a subtle way of introducing other elements of yoga such as the chakras, which each have their unique colour and emotional significance. Meditation is introduced in a very basic way as they sit listening to the sounds outside – often only the odd bird tweeting.

➤ AGES NINE TO TWELVE:
stretching as they grow

Classes for this age take into account the fact that children are very tired. They come after school, having already done an hour's homework, and are quite often on their mobile phones when they arrive. They may be exhausted from hormonal changes and the increased pressure at school. Their world is very instant, without much groundedness. We give them take-home tools to manage their stresses. If they are physically tired, they are shown a gentle energising backbend over a bolster. If they are mentally exhausted, the humming bee

breath is superb for clearing the mind.

Children of this age often aren't as flexible as we think. They are doing a huge amount of growing. Their bones grow more quickly than their muscles, making the muscles relatively shorter and less flexible.

Children also spend more time sitting on chairs at school and hunched over homework. This shortens the hip flexor muscles and creates tension in the upper back and shoulders. Postures to counteract this include stirring the pot (like 'magic pot', page 71, but without the magic element this time), side stretches and shoulder exercises. We also loosen up the wrists to prevent repetitive strain injury (RSI) which can occur from hours of writing and computer use. They now have sufficient strength to tackle sun salutations and arm balances such as crow and handstand, which gives them confidence in an environment that's still very playful.

They are fascinated by the esoteric aspects of yoga and love what they see as the 'freakiness' of it. They are very open to colour visualisations (as on page 68) only now they use words such as 'courageous' and 'free' to describe how they feel.

➤ AGE THIRTEEN UPWARDS:
body confidence and grounding

Teenagers suffer greatly from shoulder tension as a result of hunching over desks and carrying heavy school bags. Developing girls can be self-conscious about their breasts and often fold their arms in front, which rounds the shoulders. Side stretches, shoulder shrugging and heart-opening postures, such as backbends, help release tension and increase body confidence. Sun salutations exhaust them but are so good for flexibility, strength and stamina. Inversions,

such as handstand and headstand, combat mental fatigue, increase confidence and relieve tired and aching growing legs. Inversions come into their own at exam time because they are energising and brain-boosting as well as calming and meditative.

Most of the time it's visualisation and restorative poses that they really want. The pressure at school and the curveballs thrown by their hormones are even more intense now. Teenagers are very internal, working out who they are and what to do with their life. There's a lot of free-floating anxiety and so they need time to find some inner groundedness. They feel safe talking to me about being bullied at school or not having any friends. I don't offer counselling but they often feel better by being listened to and I remind them that in yoga we're all friends and everyone is doing really well.

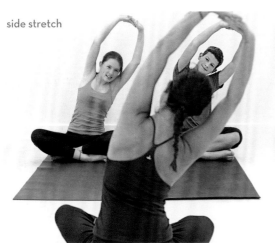

side stretch

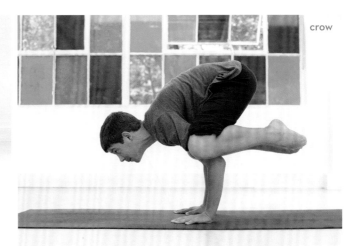

crow

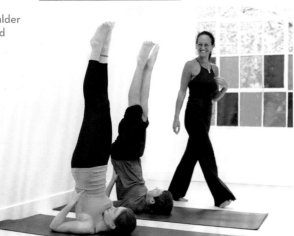

shoulder stand

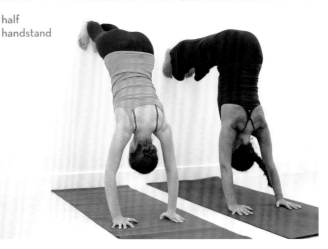

half handstand

⏰ *if you only have ten minutes*

Age seven and under: MAGIC POT

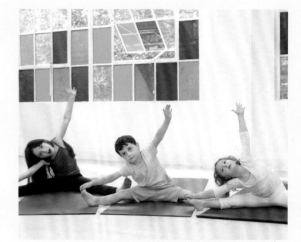

Sit with your legs wide and imagine that on the floor in front of you is a big magic pot. Reach up to the sky and take a magic ingredient – spiders, rainbows, bananas...anything! – and put it as far into the pot as you can reach, using alternate arms first and then both, but keeping your bottom on the floor. Stir as wide a circle as you can five times in each direction. Then reach far inside the pot, grab some of the magic and eat it up, keeping your bottom on the floor. Reach both arms into the sky, and then reach for your toes.

Age eight and upwards:
HUMMING BEE BREATH

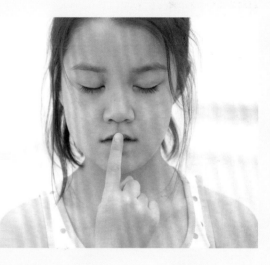

Sit comfortably and take a long, deep breath in through the nose, placing a finger on your lips, which should be lightly touching, with the teeth slightly apart. Exhale, making a humming sound through your lips. You should feel a tingling sensation on your finger. Remove your finger and close your ears with your hands and repeat. It should sound like a bee is flying around inside your head. Repeat with the hands resting by your sides.

The adult counts the child's breath (faster for younger children to give them a greater sense of achievement). Count in real-time seconds once they reach age nine. See if they can increase their count each time.

This is especially good for teens as it helps relieve mental fog and tiredness as well as clearing the mind when studying for exams.

Teens: LEGS-UP-THE-WALL POSE

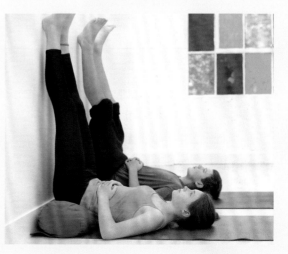

This soothes growing legs, refreshes a tired mind and calms the nervous system. Do it before bed and at exam time.

Lie on your back with your bottom close to the wall, legs extending straight up. Place a bolster or a couple of cushions under the hips. If straightening your legs is difficult, come away from the wall a little and bend them. Lie with eyes closed and hands by your sides for a few minutes. Come down if you start to lose sensation in the legs.

pregnancy yoga

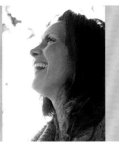

A supportive and informative practice of poses, breathing exercises and meditation to strengthen body and mind in preparation for labour and motherhood. Suitable from the second trimester

BY NADIA NARAIN

➤ MY LIGHTBULB MOMENT

When I was 18 and living in LA a friend took me to my first yoga class at the house of Kundalini yoga teacher Gurmukh Kaur Khalsa. Gurmukh also taught pregnancy yoga and I was struck by how radiant her students looked. I wasn't interested in teaching yoga, never mind pregnancy yoga, but in her and what she was doing, so I began to sit in on class. The way she talked about pregnancy was different from anything I had heard. It wasn't a scary experience which you had to numb yourself from. She empowered women; they walked out feeling great about themselves. When she created a teacher-training course, I took it and then assisted her in training others.

➤ IT'S NATURAL TO BE AFRAID

Women can be very scared of their body changing, and of labour. They hear so much that's negative about birth, so it can come as a surprise when they attend a pregnancy yoga class and find someone talking positively and honestly about what they are going through. I invite women to come back to class and tell their birth stories and I read out emails that they have sent me, asking me to pass on their advice and experiences.

I want women to come away from class saying, 'Yes, my baby is growing inside me, and it's great!' as opposed to 'I feel so big and horrible and I can't fit into my jeans.' And that goes for labour too. What if you tweaked your perspective, and, rather than thinking, 'It's going to be screaming agony, I won't be able to cope,' how about welcoming each contraction as a step closer to meeting your baby?

➤ PREGNANCY YOGA IS A TIME TO CONNECT WITH YOUR BABY

Women who are working during pregnancy don't often have the opportunity to connect with their unborn baby. The office environment makes almost no concessions to pregnancy. Women are expected to behave as if nothing had changed. Even if they are not working, if it's their second or third baby, they often simply don't have time.

I ask women to put their hands on their baby at any opportunity. I use words to connect them to their body,

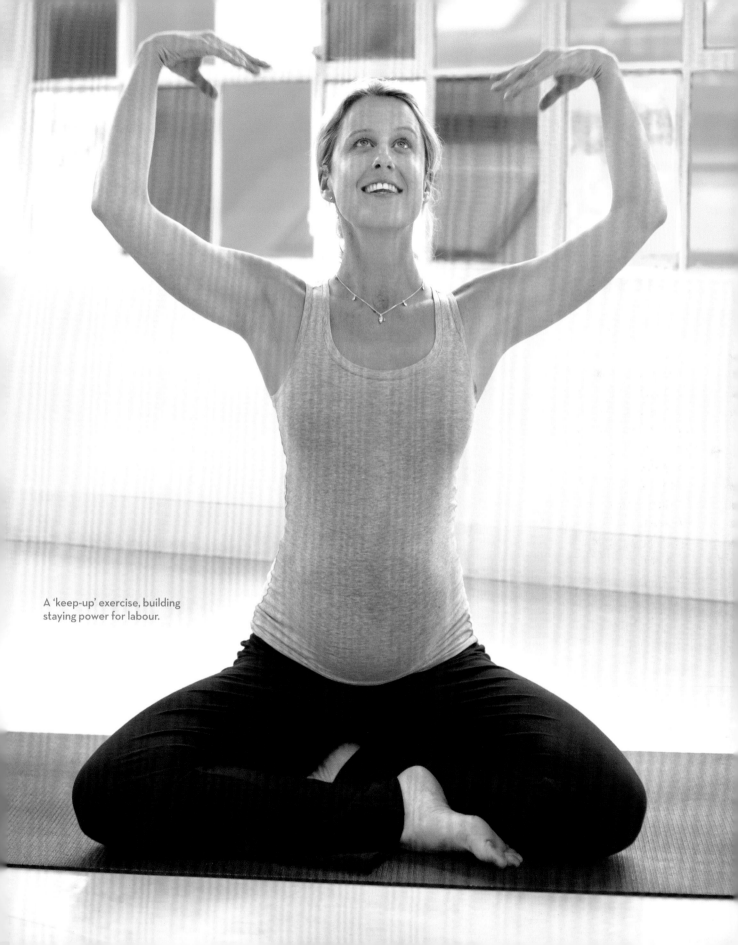

A 'keep-up' exercise, building staying power for labour.

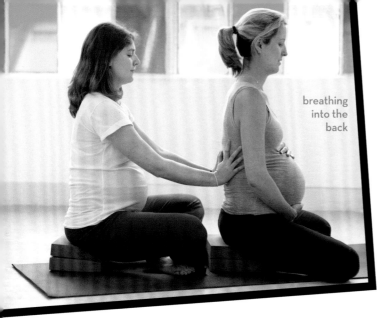

breathing into the back

their baby and their breath. For some this comes naturally, but for others it feels foreign. But in those 40 weeks of pregnancy you are never more connected to your baby.

It's also a time to connect with other pregnant women and feel part of a community, to exchange views, make friends, and to turn a unique, potentially isolating experience into a shared one.

➤ WE START WITH BREATHING EXERCISES

In pregnancy there's so much going on that women need to take deeper, fuller breaths to keep body and mind calm and steady. As the baby grows, there's less space for the lungs to expand and women find themselves short of breath. Developing awareness of posture and practising movements to lengthen the body help create as much space as possible for the woman and her baby.

The breath is key to staying present during labour as well as to staying centred when the aspects of life that we can't control – an interfering mother-in-law or changes at work – threaten to throw us off balance. I start the class by asking women to rest their hands on their belly and to feel and deepen their breath.

➤ BALANCING STRENGTH WITH SOFTNESS

We work on strengthening arms and legs, moving into different positions and working with gravity so that

women discover what their changing body is capable of. Many women say to me, 'I didn't know I could do so much.' While women need every part of their body to be strong in labour, I try to encourage them to soften their belly. Women who have high-powered jobs, or who are very strong and tight from years of gym work or dynamic yoga practice, need to spend more time softening and letting go. Holding everything in creates tension, which is not helpful in labour. I try to create a balance between being strong and soft.

➤ THEN WE WORK ON MENTAL STRENGTH

By using three-minute 'keep-up' exercises (which I learned from Gurmukh) I teach women to build mental and emotional strength in the face of discomfort. This is a mindset they will need one hundred-fold during labour. For example, while sitting we reach our arms overhead and shake the wrists vigorously as if shaking off water. It acts as a letting-go, shaking out fears. After a while, your arms really ache, so much so that your mind wants to pull you out of that situation (as it will in the pain of labour). But the challenge is to stay with it. Each week I see women build strength and staying power. Everyone groans when we do these exercises, but they feel hugely empowered when they manage the full three minutes.

➤ MEDITATION AND RELAXATION

There's so much pressure to stay on top of everything, even when you are pregnant and the body is working for two. Relaxation at the end of class allows women to rest, even for a few minutes. Meditation practices are very helpful to steady the mind and keep the nervous system calm – powerful techniques to develop in preparation for motherhood.

➤ IT'S ALL IN THE PREPARATION

Giving birth is like any big physical and mental challenge in life: you have to prepare. Your body is doing the most difficult thing it is ever going to do. Treat your birth like you would your wedding, the most important job application of your life or running a marathon. You wouldn't breeze through any of these events without preparation, hoping that things will somehow be OK.

Pregnancy is a time to get your head around the fact that the birth is going to be intense, painful for some, beautiful, magical and powerful, and to learn strategies – especially breathing deeply – to get through it. In a marathon, there's a point at which you 'hit the wall', and want to give up. It's the same in labour, at 'transition', which occurs between the contraction phase and the pushing stage. The baby is about to come out, the whole body is opening up. Even if you had planned a natural birth, that's the time when you usually call for the drugs. But if you understand what is going on in the body and can breathe into it and open up to it, you have more options.

➤ KNOWLEDGE IS POWER

It's lovely when a woman comes into class never intending to have a natural birth – in fact, is quite fixed on an epidural or a C-section – and slowly, week by week, she starts to enquire about other options. Some women have never entertained the idea of taking a more active role in their birth; perhaps out of fear or because they simply didn't know that they could. The more educated you become, the stronger you feel, so you are not just handing the experience over to someone else. Being informed also helps you to accept any medical decisions that need to be made because you have questioned them and understand them.

➤ IF YOU HAVE PLANNED A C-SECTION, PREGNANCY YOGA IS STILL FOR YOU

Students who have had C-sections report that having done pregnancy yoga makes a phenomenal difference to their healing. It helps keep your body strong and your circulation functioning well, so that you recover better. There are very few reasons why you can't come to yoga if you are pregnant, although if you have a medical condition, always check with your doctor. You could still come to class after your first trimester just to be with other women and listen to what's being said. I have had women in my classes who have only ever done the keep-up exercises or singing the prayer to the baby.

if you only have ten minutes

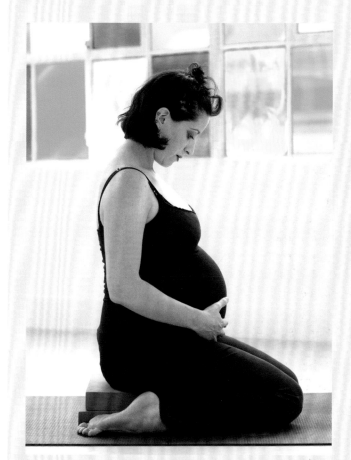

PUT YOUR HANDS ON YOUR BABY

Come on to your hands and knees and rotate the pelvis. Tilt it back and forth. This is helpful if you have back pain, plus it's a powerful position to use in labour.

Then sit with your hands on your baby. As you breathe in, feel your belly moving into the palms of your hands, and as you breathe out, feel your belly releasing towards you, keeping it soft and relaxed.

Talk to your baby. You might have had an argument with your husband or a bad day at work, but it's really nice just to sit there with your hands on your belly and say, 'That was a bad day today, but I am so happy that you are here and I can't wait to meet you.' Share a little bit of each day with your baby.

restorative yoga

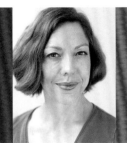

A passive, calm, restful class
to counteract stress and
rejuvenate body and mind

BY ANNA ASHBY

➤ MY LIGHTBULB MOMENT

I was 19, that precarious age where you don't know
who you are or quite what you are going to do with your
life. I was anxious and full of self-doubt. As a dancer and
performer, I was constantly comparing myself with
others, which created a lot of suffering for me. Nothing
directed me back to myself or encouraged me to settle
into my own skin. Then my best friend introduced me
to yoga through a meditation intensive. My life totally
rearranged itself from the inside out. I stopped looking
outside for security and directed my attention inwards.
Learning that 'God' was actually an expression of my
own consciousness, and that this consciousness
expressed itself through everybody, made sense to me.
I moved to an ashram – a yoga community – in New
York. Learning more about yoga teachings and
practices there was the best way to spend my twenties.
I ended up staying for 12 years.

➤ RESTORATIVE YOGA IS QUIET, RESTFUL AND HEALING

We rest in supported positions over bolsters and
blankets in order to allow the body to open, the breath
to deepen and the nervous system to slow down. The
eyes are closed and the focus is inwards. A class
comprises four or five poses held anywhere from five
to 15 minutes.

Even though you might experience a deep stretch in
some of the poses, there's no active engagement of the
muscles; it's all about allowing the body to soften

through complete support and conscious breath.

It's easy to think that lying down over a bolster for an
hour and a half is somehow indulgent – to the extent
that we may be reluctant to give ourselves permission
to do it. There's also the misconception that it's 'not
really yoga'. In fact, restorative yoga is immensely
powerful and to me is the closest thing to the practice
of meditation.

If you are on the go all the time and used to having
constant sensory input, simply lying down with nothing
to do can be extremely challenging. But, as with any
new practice, it's something that you cultivate over
time, and eventually you realise that you cannot live
without it.

➤ IT ACTIVATES THE 'OFF' SWITCH

This type of yoga practice engages the parasympathetic
nervous system (PNS) which slows down the body and
mind. The PNS is one of two aspects of our nervous
system – the sympathetic nervous system (SNS), which
engages the 'fight or flight' response, being the other.

The SNS is an activating system. It speeds up
brainwaves, increases both heart rate and breath and
contracts muscles so that we can respond quickly. In
order to maintain this heightened state, it reroutes
energy from systems that are, in that moment, non-
essential – the reproductive system, the digestive
system and the immune system. Digestion especially
becomes affected when we are under stress. Stress is
one of the biggest contributory factors to illness.

Because our attention is constantly being drawn in by emails, TV, news, the internet, mobile phones, most of us are overstimulated.

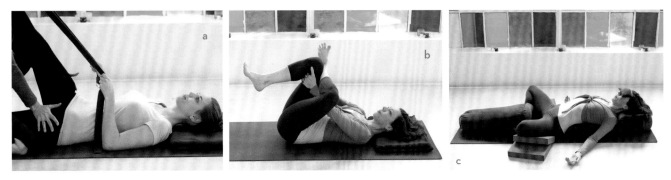

The PNS, on the other hand, is a quieting mode which puts the brakes on the activating systems and initiates a relaxation response. It slows down brainwaves, breath and heartbeat and lowers blood pressure. Restorative yoga switches off 'go' mode, allowing energy to be redirected to other systems. We may not need digestion, reproduction and so on in an acute situation, but for our wellbeing these processes are vital. When you hear your stomach gurgling in class, that's a classic indication of the PNS at work; yawning is another. If you are recovering from illness or injury, this practice won't tax the body and will support healing.

➤ IT'S THE PERFECT ANTIDOTE TO THE INFORMATION AGE

Because our attention is constantly being drawn to emails, TV, news, the internet, mobile phones and so on, most of us are overstimulated, with the result that our SNS stays stuck on 'go'. Evolution hasn't kept up with the technological age; our minds are not equipped to process such a large amount of stimulus. The result can be extreme disturbances in the mind and body that can result in conditions such as depression, anxiety and insomnia or a feeling of disconnection from the world.

When we're in a state of overstimulation, we tend to think ahead of ourselves, leaping from one thought to another or dwelling obsessively on the past. Either way we are not 'there' in the moment, present with our body and breath. When the PNS is engaged through a practice such as restorative yoga, there is a deeper breath which supports a present, calm and relaxed state. Accessing this state is something we need to experience every day as part of a balanced and healthy life, but how many of us give ourselves the time?

Physiologically, it takes anywhere from 12 to 15 minutes for the nervous system to 'gear down', which is why we stay in poses for longer periods. If you are chronically stressed it can take considerably longer to recalibrate the system.

➤ A TYPICAL CLASS INCLUDES...

We start with gentle, slow stretches **(a)**, to release tension and connect with the breath to bring the mind back into the awareness of the physical body and the present moment. I always include hip-openers, such as eye of the needle **(b)**, to open up the pelvis. If your pelvis is gripped by tight hip muscles, this can pull on the lower back. And because the first three lumbar vertebrae connect to the diaphragm, any pulling in this area will restrict the diaphragm too. The result? A more shallow breath. So when you start with gentle, slow stretches, particularly in these areas, the diaphragm can move more freely, you can breathe more deeply and this supports a parasympathetic response. Then we move into the classic restorative postures – supported backbends, forward bends, twists and inversions. Most of us are to some extent rounded in the upper body, so in class we can counteract that by lying over a bolster in a gentle supported backbend such as *supta baddha konasana* (reclining bound angle pose **(c)**). The effect is energising but still calm and easeful. Those who suffer from anxiety or an agitated mind may find supported forward bends, such as supported child's pose **(d)**, helpful as they are introspective and extremely calming. Supported twists such as *jathara parivartanasana* (revolved abdominal pose **(e)**) are powerful for releasing deep-seated muscular tension, which frees the breath, and for promoting healthy digestion. Inversions are calming and grounding. In restorative yoga we use gentle versions of

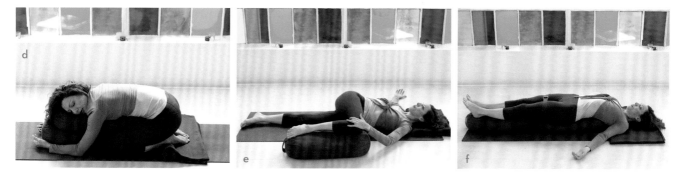

these such as bridge pose **(f)**, or legs-up-the-wall pose. Every class ends with the quintessential restorative posture of *savasana*, or corpse pose. It's here that the overall affect of the sequence takes root and the nervous system can fully rebalance.

➤ IT'S NOT SLEEP, NOR IS IT MEDITATION...

The quality of this practice is one of deep resting – more restful often than sleep. In the sleep state, the mind can be very active. Most of us know what it's like to wake up feeling like we've just been part of a high-octane action movie. Dreams can evoke a physiological response, such as tension, which stimulates the SNS. You can liken restorative yoga to 'reclining' meditation, but there's a subtle difference in intention. In meditation you are usually upright, cultivating a present state of awareness that is alert, whereas in restorative yoga your intention is to invoke a deep state of relaxation that physiologically rejuvenates the body and slows down the mind.

➤ LYING DOWN IS ALL VERY WELL, BUT WHAT ABOUT A WORKOUT?

Always balance a restorative practice with a more active one – the body and mind need both. Adding a restorative class to your weekly regime – perhaps at the end of the week when you are gearing down – can be an extremely beneficial balance to your practice. If you are doing a home practice, include a restorative pose at the end of your active practice before final relaxation (*savasana*). If you are very stressed or tired you might need to set aside the more active practice altogether for the time being in favour of a restorative one.

🕐 *if you only have ten minutes*

EFFORTLESS REST POSE

Find a quiet space where there are minimal distractions. Turn off your phone. Lie on your back with feet flat, knees bent upwards, head supported on a blanket, and hands resting on the front of your body or by your sides. Focus on relaxing the body into gravity and discovering a deeper, more easeful breath. Breathe into your centre, however you may experience that. Give your full focus to the feeling and sensation of the breath moving into your centre. This can be done in the middle of the day, at home, in a spare room at work or even in the park. If you can't find a space to lie down, simply sit upright, close the eyes, relax (particularly face and shoulders) and breathe.

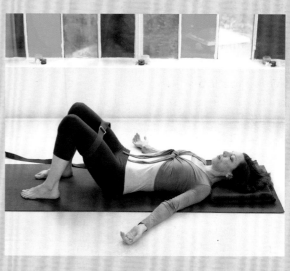

yoga for runners + sports

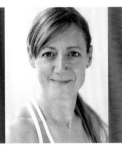

A dynamic yoga class grounded in biomechanics, sports psychology and philosophy to enhance running and sports performance, both physically and mentally – and to help practitioners enjoy their athletic potential

BY LAURA DENHAM-JONES

➤ MY LIGHTBULB MOMENT

I don't think it's an accident that the only two major sports injuries I've had – a hip injury from distance running and knee damage from cycling – happened before I did yoga. I used to do things to extremes. I'd run every day, making the runs longer and longer, and without allowing my body enough time to recover. The same applied to my work and social life. I would overcommit myself and burn out.

When I took up yoga seriously after ten years of running competitively, I was surprised to notice that I could take a couple of months off from running without any loss of fitness. Neither did I need as much recovery time between sprints in training. I also became less injury-prone – yoga made me more mindful as well as improving my strength and alignment. Previously I would have 'run through' an injury – a classic competitive athlete's thing to do, when of course that only makes it worse. The philosophy of yoga teaches you to listen to your body and be kind to it. If I ever get a little niggle now, I'll ease back and it usually goes away.

➤ YOGA HELPS YOU PACE YOURSELF

As well as listening to your body to help you decide when to work harder and when to ease back, yoga teaches you to catch any negative thoughts before you become discouraged by staying in the moment through focusing on your breath. During a marathon I used to think too often about how much of the race was left, telling myself that I could never finish at such-and-such a pace, so I might as well give up and walk. I learned that if I stayed in the present and simply put one foot in front of the other, I would soon be fine as tiredness comes in waves. I try to remind myself that these are the fluctuations of the mind and that I can transcend them. I tell myself, 'You are where you are supposed to be – focus on what you are doing right now.'

Self-acceptance, patience and staying in the present also help with competitive sports where points are scored against an opponent. Tennis players, for example, benefit greatly from the yoga mentality of letting go of outcome and staying focused on composure in action. This means not allowing the mind

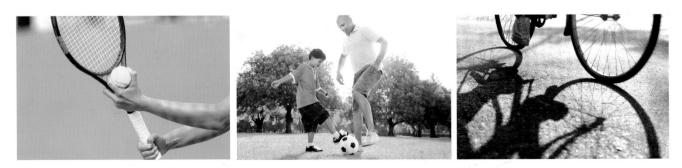

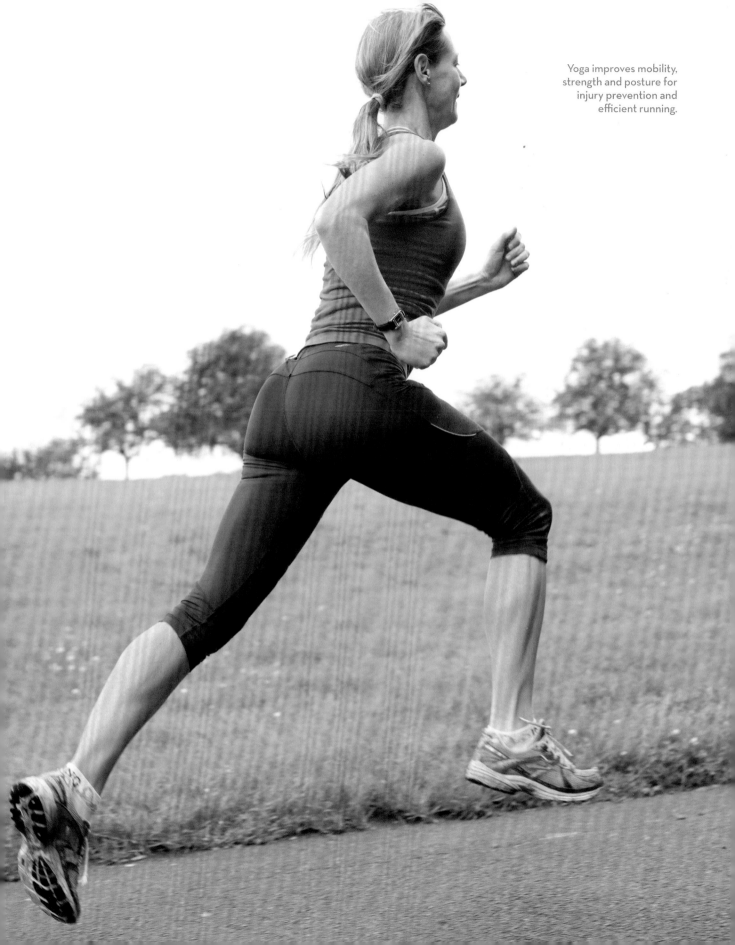

Yoga improves mobility,
strength and posture for
injury prevention and
efficient running.

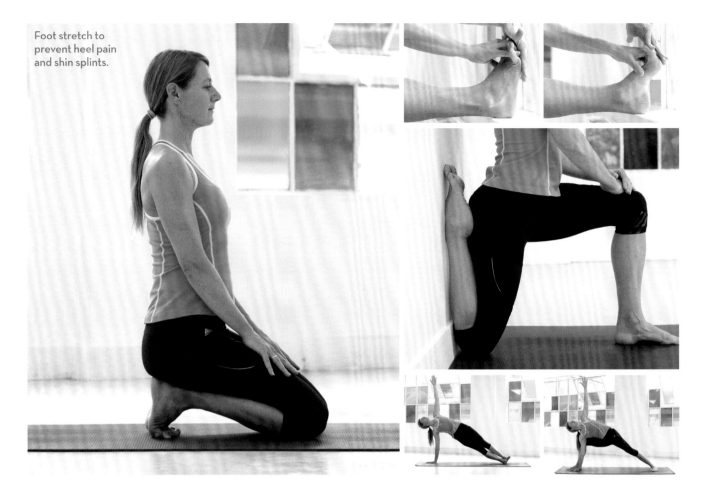

Foot stretch to prevent heel pain and shin splints.

to give up before the body does just because the momentum has shifted to the other player. It means letting go of the distracting frustrations about an umpire's decision and moving on with a clear mind. Many top tennis players, such as Andy Murray, Maria Sharapova and Rafael Nadal, practise yoga.

➤ YOGA MAKES YOU AN ALL-ROUNDER

Many athletes come to yoga for the stretch but it's obviously not all that yoga is. Aside from its philosophical aspects, the practice is about balancing out the strengths and weaknesses of the body.

Racket and hand-to-eye ball sports involve repetitive motions on one side of the body only – in yoga we work in symmetry.

In much aerobic exercise, such as running and cycling, we move mostly in one plane of motion. In yoga we use all planes of motion and movement types – forward bending, side bending, back bending, rotation,

flexion, extension, abduction and adduction – and we do this sitting, standing, supine, upside down. Few sports offer such variety. We activate muscles underused in day-to-day life and even in certain sports. We can rest or stretch muscles which are overused or tense, such as upper shoulders and hamstrings. And if it's more flexibility we're after, it's sometimes not just about stretching one muscle group, such as the hamstrings, ad nauseam. Instead, we can strengthen other muscles that might share the work with them. Weak glutes or quads might be the cause of tight hamstrings in some runners.

➤ YOGA IS NON-COMPETITIVE BUT IT HELPS YOU COMPETE IN OTHER DISCIPLINES

Yoga helps develop the mental strength to work at our threshold and to breathe through discomfort, but also the awareness not to push across the line into true

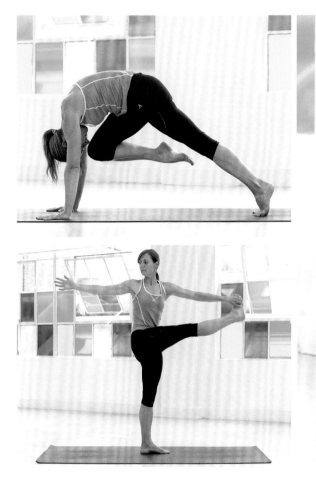

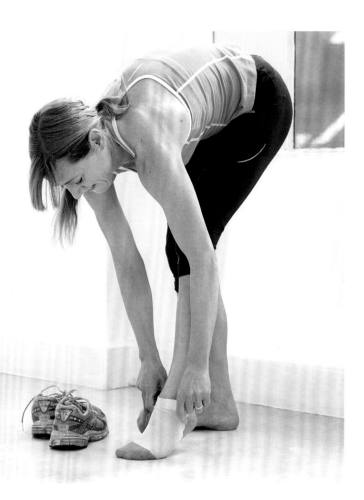

pain or illness for the sake of short-term results. Yoga techniques such as counting the breaths, or repeating a simple mantra, such as 'yes' or 'keep going', can help with the single-mindedness needed to compete or improve.

That said, it also teaches us to listen to feedback from the body to ensure that it isn't becoming a sacrifice for the end goal. Part of being a successful competitor is not taking rivalries to a personal level.

Elite athletes do sometimes have to psych themselves up about their opponent. The challenge is not letting this destroy their soul. In Andre Agassi's autobiography *Open*, he talks about the physical and mental price of competition. As a tennis pro he felt obliged to win, but unqualified for any other profession. He became trapped – pushing his body to attain victories while secretly hating the chore it had become. All this underscores the need for some kind of spiritual respite, such as yoga.

➤ IT'S ABOUT TAKING YOUR EYE *OFF* THE PRIZE

The aim of a yoga for runners and sports class is to create body awareness in a situation where the students aren't – for once – striving for a result. In a seated forward bend, for example, a goal-oriented person might try to force their head down towards their knees, hunching their spine, going for a final result (head to knees) rather than adopting a stretch that uses a smaller range of motion at first, or accepting the help of a block or belt. In that instance, I might have the whole class using props.

➤ A TYPICAL CLASS INCLUDES...

We always warm up the feet first (e.g. kneeling with toes tucked, sitting on heels), followed by sun salutations, warrior, triangle and standing balances, which create the agility needed for changing direction, running uphill or running on uneven terrain.

Dynamic flow and standing poses (especially lunges) cultivate alignment, strength and stability in the legs – especially in the knees – which are often injury-prone. The knees are slaves to the feet and pelvis. They can only do their job properly if what is above and below them is stable. So if we land our foot incorrectly when running – that is by placing too much weight on the inside or outside – or if our pelvis is uneven, it twists the knee. Simple poses such as standing with parallel feet (mountain pose) and on one leg (tree) are helpful for identifying any imbalances and correcting them.

As an athlete, you need the muscles around your ankles, knees and hips to fire quickly. In yoga we do this by shifting weight from two legs to one; such as raising one knee while standing, then shooting that leg back into lunge. Sprinters often do 'plyometrics' in training – movements which involve fast hopping and jumping. Some yoga postures offer low-impact versions of those movements, where the foot doesn't leave the floor. This is a good alternative if you have a knee or ankle injury.

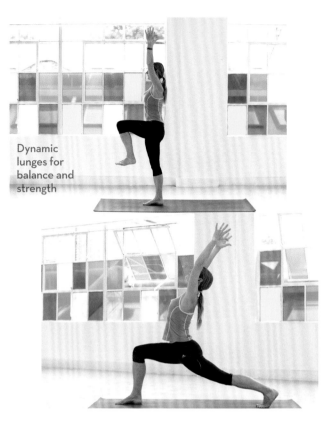

Dynamic lunges for balance and strength

DON'T IGNORE THE CORE

Strong abdominals, back and pelvic floor muscles give us a strong centre for the limbs, as levers, to pull and push from. If the lower back and hip muscles are constantly correcting alignment problems in the trunk, the body tires more quickly and injury sets in.

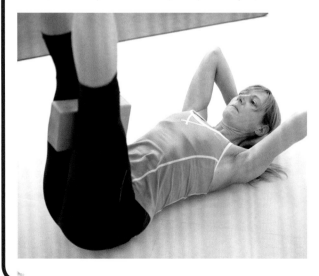

TWISTS ARE IMPORTANT TOO

When we run, one side of the pelvis comes forward with the leg along with the opposite shoulder. Passive spinal twists in yoga help loosen the muscles required for this movement, while strong twists develop strength and tone to control the necessary rotation.

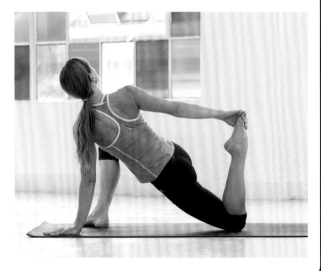

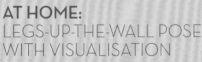 if you only have ten minutes

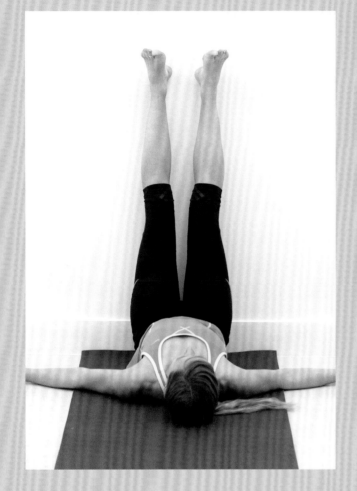

AT HOME:
LEGS-UP-THE-WALL POSE WITH VISUALISATION

Lie with your legs up the wall, close your eyes and relax. Elevating the legs – especially if you spend a lot of time on your feet – drains fluids from the tissues of the lower legs, gets lymph circulating to support the immune system and lowers heart rate and blood pressure. Use this time to examine in your mind how you are going to attempt to perform in a race or event. This takes concentration and energy, so is best done a day or so before the event, not directly before. Then take a few moments to relax.

BEFORE AND AFTER SPORT:
STANDING PIGEON OR 'FIGURE 4' POSE

I do this before and after a run. Stand with feet hip-width apart and bend the knees. Cross one ankle over the opposite thigh, near the knee. Bring your palms together at your chest and fold forwards from the hips, with a long spine, drawing your chin slightly in and resting your elbows above the knee and ankle. Hold for several breaths. As a balance, it develops focus and confidence, as well as strengthening the ankle and stretching the hip rotators that stabilise the pelvis when you are running.

Scaravelli-inspired

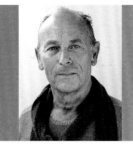

A gentle yet challenging class highlighting the deep and active movement of the spine

BY JOHN STIRK

➤ MY LIGHTBULB MOMENT

It was more like a fog lifting and it was immediate. In my twenties, I had several long-standing ailments – lower back pain, chronic bronchitis and recurrent depression. My girlfriend Lolly (now my wife), who was a yoga teacher, showed me some simple standing postures and how to use the breath to release tension and stiffness. The results were astonishing. After several weeks of daily practice – often twice or three times per day – my lower back had released, my chest began to open and I could think clearly for the first time in ages.

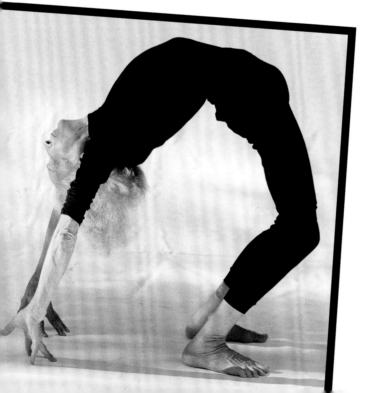

The effect on my mind was unexpected and profound. It felt as if the yoga within me had just been waiting to happen. I had to share this extraordinary discovery and the next step was to start teaching.

➤ VANDA SCARAVELLI WAS A REMARKABLE ADVERT FOR HER WORK

In 1989 I began to study with 81-year-old Vanda Scaravelli (below left), who came to yoga in her 40s under the tutelage of yoga masters BKS Iyengar and TKV Desikachar. Although she had worked with the great teachers of her time, she said that her real learning and understanding began when she stopped seeing her teachers. This gave her the opportunity for a deep and dedicated personal practice.

I was struck by the way her body – particularly her spine – responded in postures. She moved internally in a way that I had not seen before and this appealed to me as an osteopath as well as a yoga teacher. All her bones moved rhythmically from within, displaying great space and vitality. The action and release of her spine appeared to come by itself and underpinned all postures, conveying a sense of enormous freedom. She was interested in my osteopathic background. Her first words to me were, 'Hello, tell me about the cerebrospinal fluid [CSF], because I have had an elbow problem and I have managed to resolve it with the breathing.'

So I told her how the CSF bathes and nourishes the nervous system and that the osteopathic profession

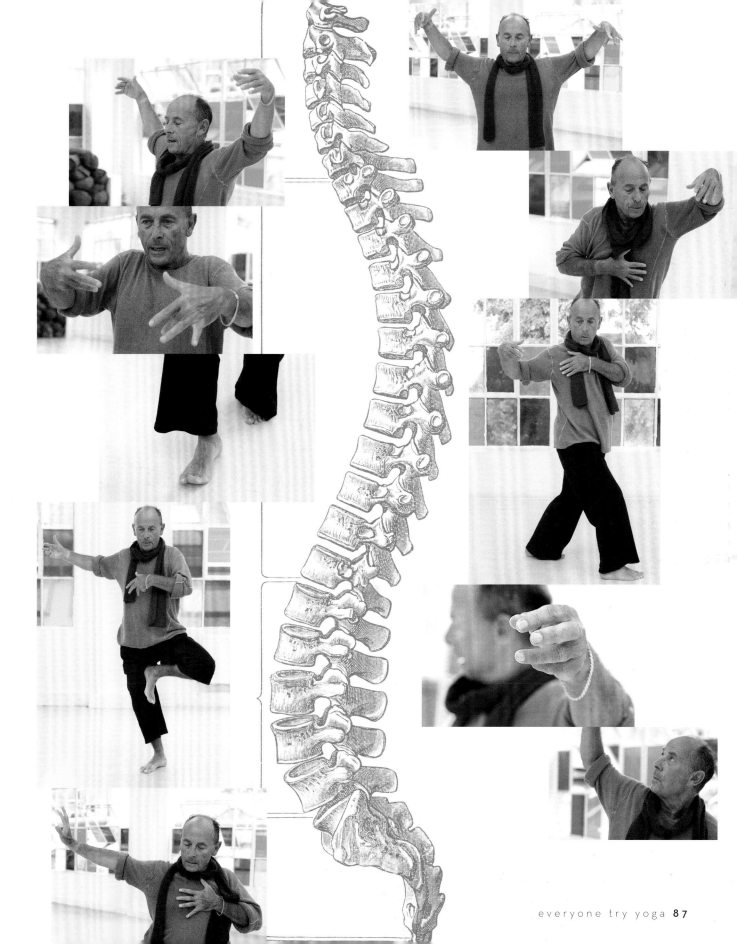

considered its unimpaired flow to be an essential factor in health and healing. Through the deep work with her breath she had probably given her elbow a surge of this fluid and helped to clear the irritation and inflammation. She began to teach me, giving her time and energy freely and generously, until shortly before her death in 1999 at the age of 91.

➤ DISSOLVING TENSION IN BODY AND MIND

The Scaravelli approach is suitable for anyone interested in awakening a deeper intelligence in order to undo tension in body and mind.

One works with the inner body and softens the outer body, always coming back to the spine. This has a powerful effect by giving us greater lightness, freedom and softness. Finding the release, natural action and intelligence takes time and work; but if one is interested it brings great rewards.

➤ SCARAVELLI TEACHERS VARY THEIR APPROACH

Vanda gave her students plenty of space to develop in their own way, leaving them free to teach their own interpretation. The common thread is how one approaches the tension or resistance encountered in the postures. The emphasis is on giving one's weight to the ground, while following the movement of the breath inside oneself. This stimulates a deep movement that begins in the spine and spreads throughout the body.

Classes are usually slow in their pace. Vanda understood the importance of not forcing or over-extending. The focus is on the quality of movement and how one is from moment to moment. This approach gives a tremendous sense of integration between body and mind. However, it brings its own challenges. You need to cultivate the art of listening to your inner voice and have an interest in dissolving your habitual patterns of physical and mental tension. Vanda was a true advocate of finding yoga in oneself and for oneself. For me this is the essential aspect of her teaching. There is no 'Scaravelli method' as such, because listening involves adjusting to the ever-changing tensions and activity in practice.

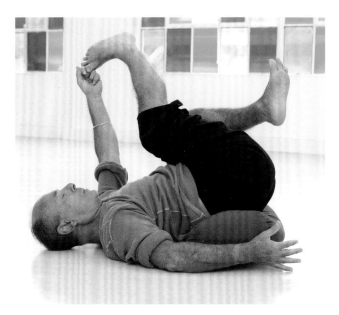

➤ THE SPINE PROVIDES THE ULTIMATE PHYSICAL YOGA EXPERIENCE

All parts of the body are in some way either directly or indirectly connected to the spine and everything we feel during practice is relayed via the spinal cord. In view of this, cultivating a practice that appeals directly to the spine is essential for maximising the benefits of yoga. The ancient yogis understood that releasing the spine's inherent energy had a direct effect on the expansion of consciousness. Science also believes that human consciousness evolved in part from energy arising from the base of the spine, moving upwards through energy centres in and around the spine, towards the brain.

The spine has enormous potential for the kind of sensitivity needed for intelligent practice. Its natural state is to respond to the downward pull of gravity by lengthening and opening. But life – with its physical and emotional pressures – has meant that we are depriving it of that ability. Yoga reawakens this function. A free spine enriches the yoga practice and enhances all the benefits that it brings.

When we focus on freeing the spine it also becomes clear that it has a wave-like motion that relates to the rhythm of the breath. This feeds into and enhances the texture of the entire body. As the spine awakens, we become more sensitive to our tensions and we can release them more easily. This is felt as a physical and mental melting of tension and resistance. We work from the spine in all postures, and yet its relevance can easily be overlooked in our eagerness to *do* the postures. The spine is most responsive to a quiet interest but will retreat when we impose our will upon it. This is why we go slowly in the postures. When the spine awakens, it is like restoring life to an ancient creature within us.

➤ STUDENTS BECOME CALMER, SOFTER – AND, OCCASIONALLY, EVEN HEALED

Through such practice, students become much more physically grounded. Their upper bodies become lighter and freer and their spines spontaneously lengthen, becoming more vital in response to the breath and gravitational pull. The entire body appears more alive and inter-responsive, all parts contributing to a kind of inner dance. I notice more internal fluidity, space and softness. Students become calmer and less ruled by their emotions. They also report that their thoughts have a lighter and softer quality and they have more patience.

From time to time spontaneous healing occurs. It is not uncommon for back pain, blood-pressure imbalances, indigestion, constipation or menstrual disorders to resolve and occasionally infertility has been addressed through the practice. Most noticeable is a shared loving kindness which emerges within classes and extends well beyond the mat and into life; a healing of the spirit.

➤ WHEN THE PRACTICE BECOMES A MEDITATION

The yoga postures present ever-changing, moment-to-moment sensations. These sensations keep us right there, are in time with time, and as such provide an ideal meditation. Body and mind merge in a way that releases us from habitual mental turbulence. This gives us a basis for how to proceed both on and off the mat. The calm lightness and freedom from habit experienced in practice gives us a benchmark for an alternative way of being in life generally. The inherent intelligence of the body/mind recognises a good thing when it feels it, and the effects extend into daily life. This becomes a practice in itself, the practice of yoga.

⏱ *if you only have ten minutes*

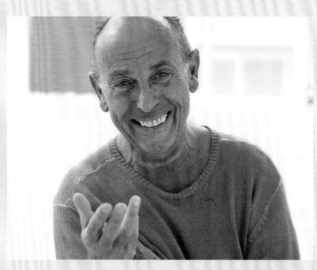

IT IS NOT SO MUCH ABOUT WHICH POSTURE TO DO, BUT ABOUT HOW ONE IS WITHIN THE POSTURE

Choose a few simple postures that you are familiar with and that provide just enough resistance to work with – and remember to stay relaxed.

From there, work deeply inside yourself and look for a pause that takes place at the end of each exhalation. During this pause, an inner space opens up and this is the preparation for the next inhalation. Don't rush the in-breath, but allow it to arise from within you. Treat it gently; let it come by itself. Sometimes it comes immediately as a continuation of the exhalation and sometimes it may take more time to arrive. Become more sensitive to the potential lightness and freedom of your breath and you will discover the deep relationship between it, your spine and the posture. When you have to act, remain centred and well in contact with the ground. Don't be too attached to the practice. Perceive your actions and responses from a distance and soften your awareness. Allow all the sensations to pass through you; don't think too much, and give your mind's natural fluidity back to itself. Literally undo all aspects of yourself; feel free.

vinyasa flow

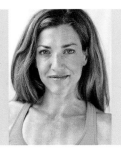

A dynamic, flowing class evolved from Ashtanga where movement is synchronised with breath

BY AMME POULTON

➤ MY LIGHTBULB MOMENT

I came into yoga for the most non-spiritual reasons. I had torn the ligaments in both knees playing soccer, and by the time I was in law school my knees were falling apart, not to mention my back, hips and shoulders! I needed to find a form of exercise I could do that was low-impact. I went to hatha yoga classes initially, but finding a modified Ashtanga class (my first experience of vinyasa flow) was when it really fell in to place. I was hooked. My teacher, Larry Schulz, picked me out early on, and with a big smile told me to 'get in the front row'. He also told me that yoga would 'ruin my life', and in a sense it did. It ruined the life I thought I was supposed to have: I was married and a corporate lawyer. Through regular practice I noticed inconsistencies in my life. Once you get into yoga, the areas where you are not in the flow start to stand out. So aged 29 I quit practising law, got divorced and started my life from scratch in a tiny studio apartment, teaching yoga. Yoga allowed me to listen to my inner voice when everyone else in the world was telling me to follow a different path.

➤ HOW FLOW HELPS YOU SLOW

When I started yoga I was beyond hyper – even my teacher told me that I twitched a lot. Slowing down was, and still is, a challenge. The physically demanding aspects of a dynamic practice allowed me to detach from my overactive and sometimes unhealthy mind and sit comfortably in my body. Once the practice got me

to this quiet place, meditation was effortless. It felt like I was tapping into a wisdom that I had spent years of my life studying in books.

It can be hard to control a busy mind if you start by sitting. The changing postures of vinyasa flow require absolute concentration. Finding a style of yoga that involves movement has meant that I can now sit still. I'm calmer, more at ease and less clumsy. It has also given me greater structural stability around my injuries.

➤ VINYASA FLOW IS ALL ABOUT...

This style of yoga synchronises your movement with your breath, building heat via sequences called *vinyasas* – mini sun salutations – which are interspersed between postures to keep the muscles warm. It's an evolution of Ashtanga, which is the archetypal vinyasa flow.

Unlike Ashtanga there is no set sequence, but that doesn't mean that we just throw postures in at random. Each pose builds on the previous one to open the body in a safe way, so that when we come to the deep or challenging postures, such as crow or handstand, the body has the strength and openness it needs to do the posture without injury. For example, to open up the flexibility of your spine you must open the muscles that connect the spine to the legs and hips first. So to build up to full wheel (see right) we'd do lunges for the front of the legs as well as hip openers such as pigeon, and then several gentler backbends such as locust and bow, all the time keeping the body warm with *vinyasas*.

eight angle pose
(*astavakrasana*)

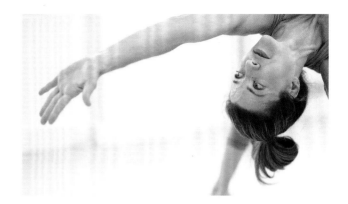

upward facing bow
(*urdhva dhanurasana*)
or wheel

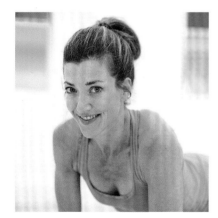

one-legged king
pigeon (*eka pada
rajakapotasana*)
variation

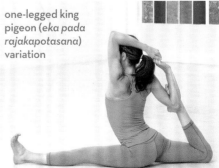

wild thing
(*camatkarasana*)

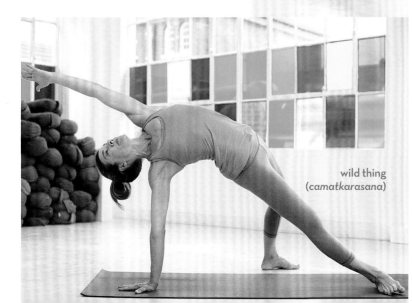

➤ BREATH + MOVEMENT = FLOW

In vinyasa flow each movement is initiated on an inhale or an exhale and we generally use *ujjayi* breath (page 168) because it creates heat and it makes a sound which is louder than your thoughts, giving you something to focus on. In yoga we want to get the breath moving deeply and evenly to calm the mind. It's often easier to ask students to get their breath moving when their body is moving also – which is the heart of vinyasa flow. Essentially it's a moving meditation.

➤ TO TRAVEL IS MORE IMPORTANT THAN TO ARRIVE

Flowing transitions between postures are as important as the postures themselves. When people tell me after class that they feel 'sore after all that stretching', I know that they've been concentrating too much on how a pose should look – gripping too tightly and jamming themselves into a particular shape – rather than how they got there. Gradually they learn to get away from the 'Am I doing it right? Where am I supposed to be?' mentality and to experience what it *feels* like in a posture. This is where the idea of flow can really help. I encourage students to feel movement even when they are still, by connecting to breath rising and falling like a wave. This generates a softness. The muscles can then release instead of resist and the body develops the 'bamboo' quality of being strong without being rigid.

A dynamic style such as this does attract the go-getting, perfectionist type-A personality. If I could tell them one thing, it would be, 'Relax already'. I always throw in one big challenging posture so that students learn that it's OK not to have it work out. Their challenge is to maintain their mental equilibrium in that situation. I remind them that the sign that their yoga is advancing is not whether they can 'do' every pose, but can they breathe in every pose?

➤ WHAT ABOUT ALIGNMENT?

It's often said that 'there's no alignment in vinyasa flow'. True: you don't stay in any one pose long enough to focus in depth. But alignment is something that you can develop in your practice when you use the breath as a tool. By studying the changes in your breath as you travel through different postures – is it shallow, are you panting, is the inhale shorter than the exhale? – you learn to make adjustments in your alignment so that you can breathe deeply and evenly.

➤ TO GROOVE OR NOT TO GROOVE?

Music is very common in dynamic classes and in the yoga community it's controversial. In a music-free class it's much easier to learn the breath because you can hear yourself and those around you. But it took me six years before I would happily go to a class without music because my mind would wander too much. My mantra is do whatever it takes to get on the mat. At home I don't use music unless I am having a sluggish day, when I'll put on some house beats to keep me going or some songs that I like to sing along to. Singing is basically *pranayama* exercise.

➤ I BALANCE MY PRACTICE WITH...

Yoga nidra, a deep, guided relaxation/meditation using a *sankalpa* (a resolve or intention) as the focus. It can be anything that is phrased in simple and positive terms – for example, 'I am... happy, healthy, joyful, aware, contented.' I have a couple of recordings that I never tire of listening to.

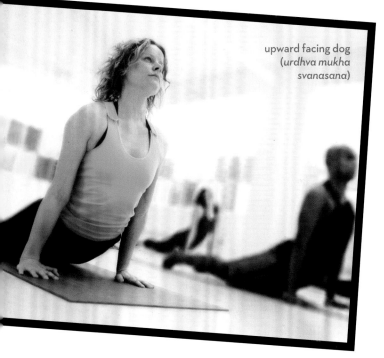

upward facing dog
(*urdhva mukha svanasana*)

⏰ *if you only have ten minutes*

My teacher always said, 'Get your head below your heart every day.' Not only does it release the weight of the head, but it also allows you symbolically to let go of anything that has been weighing heavily on the mind. When the mind is no longer heavy, the heart can be lighter and fuller. It's also a great pick-me-up. The stimulation of blood going to the head can help you feel more clear headed and alert.

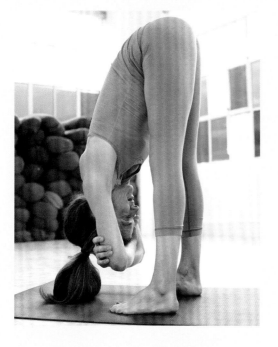

RAG DOLL

If I need a quick fix, I go straight to this modified standing forward bend (*uttanasana*). With your feet apart, knees slightly bent, hold opposite elbows with the hands. This has the added benefit of stretching the legs and back.

HANDSTAND

This is the pose I always come back to for mental focus. If you can't focus your mind no amount of physical strength will keep you up in this pose. Although it took me years to get to this place, I can now quickly bring my mind into a more settled state just by doing a quick handstand. It helps to learn it in stages below.

1. 'Upside-down handstand'. Stand upright, reaching your arms over your head while rising up on your toes. It's a lot harder than you think. You have to hug the muscles of your inner thighs towards each other, draw inwards and up with your belly (*uddiyana bandha*) and focus your eyes on one point (*drsti*). Of course, you need to breathe.

2. Downward facing dog with feet up against the wall. With your back to the wall in downward facing dog (see page 154), slowly walk your legs up to hip height, staying strong in the core to support the back.

3. Kicking up using the wall for balance. Start in downward facing dog, facing the wall this time, with your hands 30cm (1ft) away from the wall. Walk your feet in a few inches, lift one leg in the air and push up from the other.

4. Free-standing. Stay at the wall but move your hands about 45cm (1½ft) away. Keep your gaze forwards on the skirting board, take one leg up as if it were suspended by the big toe and press up from the foot on the ground. Bend one leg and place that foot on the wall, while reaching up through the other leg. When the leg in the air is strong, lift the other leg.

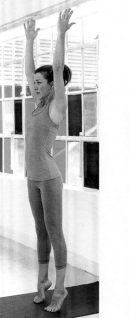
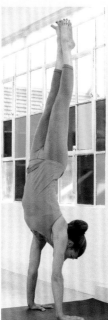

Yin

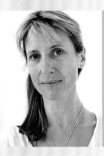

Long-held, floor-based stretches to release tension patterns, improve joint health and provide an entry point to meditation

BY JANE KERSEL

➤ MY LIGHTBULB MOMENT

I'd describe it more as natural unfolding. I had practised dynamic yoga for many years and struggled to sit in meditation for long periods as the doing/achieving parts of me felt it was a waste of time. In Yin I found a passive style where I felt comfortable enough to stay sitting, because the postures gave my 'doing mind' something to achieve. It was also a style of yoga that I could use alongside my psychological and spiritual (psycho-spiritual) studies. My Yin practice gave me the opportunity to sit with my feelings and to acknowledge them. I would be in a challenging hip opener, for example, and out of nowhere I would feel myself becoming angry and find that I was clenching my jaw. This also seemed to trigger dreams of anguish and release, and to mirror the times in my life when I was most trying to 'hold it together' externally. Yin doesn't always bring up such intense emotion or that depth of self-enquiry, but when things are chaotic off your mat it's a good place to step out of the chaos and unwind, and in that unwinding to get in touch with your vulnerability and to be OK with it.

➤ IT'S ALL ABOUT LETTING GO

Yin is a powerful way of surrendering – physically and psychologically. It is a more passive form of yoga where you spend three to five minutes in poses, which are mostly seated or lying down. They include half pigeon (page 97), seated forward bends, passive backbends such as *supta baddha konasana* (lying-down butterfly, page 96) and sphinx, deep supported lunges, *viparita karani* (legs-up-the-wall) and so on. We try to switch off the superficial muscular activity around a particular joint – sometimes using props – in order to let the deepest muscles and connective tissue release.

➤ WORKING INTO THE JOINTS

With the emphasis on muscles in most forms of exercise – including yoga *asana* practice – most of us have never given much thought to what and where our connective tissue may be.

Ligaments (which connect bone to bone) and tendons (connecting muscle to bone) are made of connective tissue. Unlike muscle, which is elastic and stretchy, connective tissue is more plastic and needs

Because Yin is passive and rejuvenating for the nervous system, it is also fantastic for people who are stressed, have adrenal burnout or chronic fatigue.

deep lunge

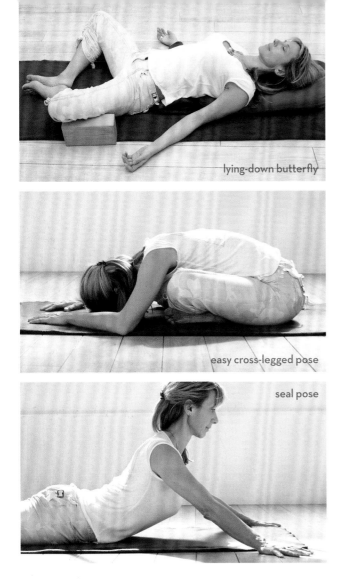

lying-down butterfly

easy cross-legged pose

seal pose

warmth and time to become more pliable – hence the reason why we stay in poses longer. Yin yoga can create more space in the joints and increase their range of motion, while keeping them healthy. Releasing the connective tissue in the hips in half pigeon, for example, can help your range of movement in other poses.

Connective tissue also wraps around every muscle and organ in the body like a huge knitted garment. If you are in a deep passive lunge, for example, you may feel the sole of your back foot become cramped or a release in your neck and shoulders. The stretch draws out the tension as if you are stretching apart a woolly jumper after it has shrunk in the wash. When one part is gently stretched it can have a profound knock-on effect throughout the body.

➤ BE CAREFUL IF YOU ARE NATURALLY VERY FLEXIBLE

There's a danger you could overstretch the joints in a Yin practice if your muscles/ligaments/tendons are naturally very flexible. Make sure you work more dynamically, activating the muscles a little so you feel your bones locating deep into your joints while in the stretch, rather than just flopping into poses.

➤ YIN YOGA WORKS ON AN ENERGETIC LEVEL TOO

Yin yoga in the form it's seen today was developed by yoga anatomy specialist Paul Grilley and is a combination of Indian yoga and Chinese Taoist philosophy. Taoism gives us the concept of *yin* (passive, deep, reflective, feminine) and *yang* (active, superficial, masculine). Many schools of yoga as well as Taoism believe in the idea of energy channels (*nadis* in yoga, *meridians* in Taoism) along which vital life force (*prana* or *chi*) flows and gathers at key centres in the body (chakras, see page 172). It's thought that these energy channels are located in the connective tissue and research by Dr Hiroshi Motoyama and others is now validating this.

In more esoteric yoga terminology, Yin works on an energetic level, stimulating the flow of *prana* in the *nadis*. As *prana* often becomes stuck in the joints (where so much meets, particularly in the hips, neck and shoulders), Yin yoga is a powerful way to shift those energy blockages.

In meridian theory, energy channels relate to the health of specific organs, so depending on the teacher you might do a sequence that works on the heart, the liver or kidney meridians. (Don't be surprised if you've worked on the kidney meridian and need to pee a lot after class!)

All Yin yoga teachers teach in their own way – some from an anatomy/physiology stance, some from a Buddhist stance, some with emphasis on cranio-sacral principles. My emphasis is psycho-spiritual and energetic and I use a process called *The Psychology of the Selves* to work through the strong feelings that Yin poses can bring out.

➤ YIN IS A GOOD COUNTERBALANCE TO A DYNAMIC (YANG) PRACTICE

If you are very stressed or exhausted, a dynamic hatha yoga class may not reduce your stress, particularly if the poses you do are challenging. If you have had an argument with your best friend, for example, a dynamic class might help you release a build-up of tension and emotion but it won't necessarily give you the space or time to reflect. A quiet, self-reflective class will drop you down into a place where you can be aware of what was really going on for you and, if need be, make changes.

I occasionally teach a course called 'Stop the world I want to get off', which is full of Yin poses. It always sells out, partly because people living in a high-octane urban environment need to be given permission to stop. If you allow yourself to let go very deeply, you might notice that you are more tired than you realised.

Because Yin is passive and rejuvenating for the nervous system, it is also fantastic for people who are stressed, have adrenal burnout or chronic fatigue.

➤ IF YOU FIND IT HARD TO SWITCH OFF, YIN CAN BE A WAY INTO MEDITATION

Yin yoga teaches you the practice of concentration, which is the first stage of meditation. In this style of yoga you are not being asked to sit up straight for meditation, which many of us find challenging. Instead, by changing position every few minutes and bringing your focus internally to a different part of you, you are deepening your self-awareness. After a while, a restlessness or boredom may start to arise. Yin yoga asks you to feel what's going on and not to go anywhere with that. If you become uncomfortable in the hips after a couple of minutes in half pigeon, for example, you may want to remove yourself from the sensations by thinking about what you're going to do later or by coming out of the pose. It teaches the practice of mindfulness meditation – sitting with what is currently present in you, without trying to change it. Once you start to notice the strategies you use to relieve boredom or discomfort on the mat, you may notice those same strategies coming up in everyday life: 'Do I not follow through in things?' 'Do I walk away when situations get uncomfortable?'

🕐 *if you only have ten minutes*

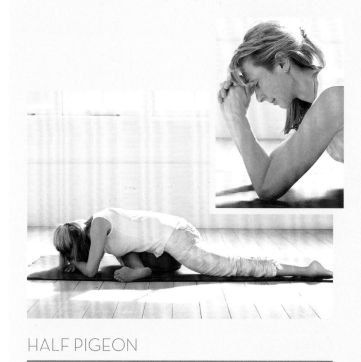

HALF PIGEON

Half pigeon is particularly beneficial if you have been sitting all day and your buttocks or hips are tight.

With the right leg forward, as shown above, place a bolster under your right sitting bone so you are slightly elevated, avoiding pressure on your knee joint. Fold forwards, resting the forehead in your hands. Feel your weight equally in the legs rather than it falling forwards.

If you have a headache, bring your elbows to the floor. Place the thumbs into the upper part of the inner eye sockets, as shown above. Rest your head on your thumbs and use that as a pressure point.

Breathe into the sensation in your eye sockets, hips and buttocks, and as you breathe out feel tension leaving like a grey smog. Keep breathing into that sensation, releasing into it, surrendering to it. You'll begin to notice the tension releasing and the mind letting go of the need to make it 'mean' something. It becomes just a sensation and in that simple act comes so much self-knowledge and maturity.

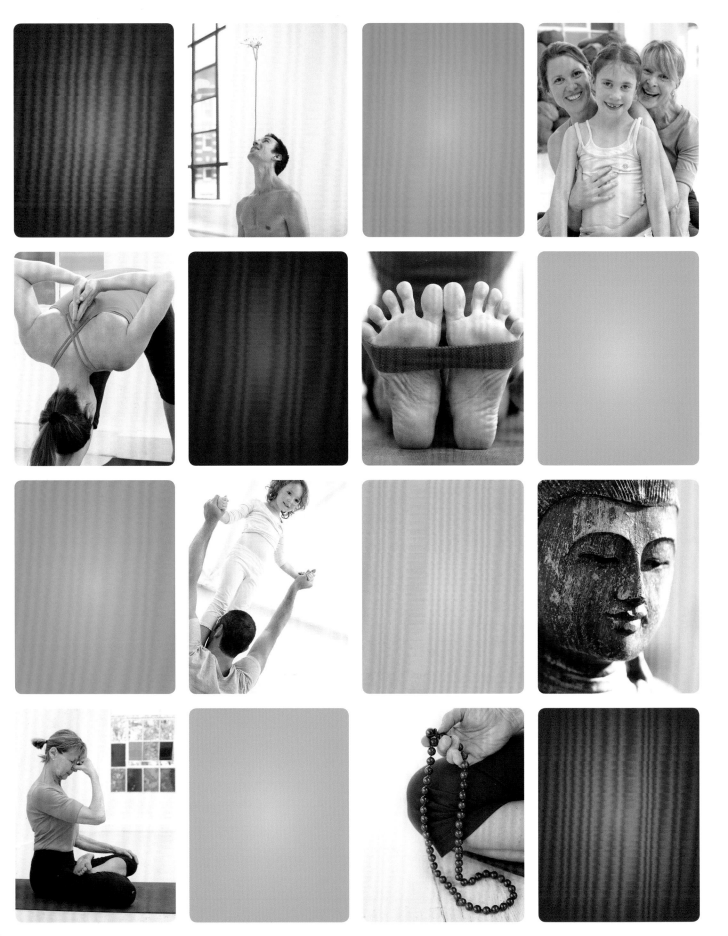

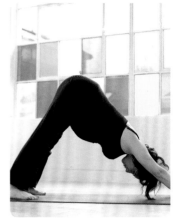

what can it do for me?

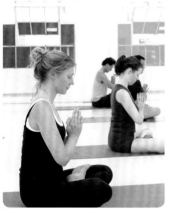
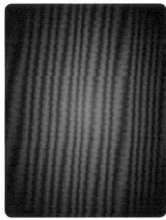
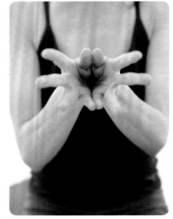
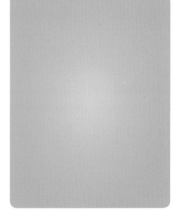

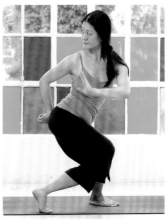

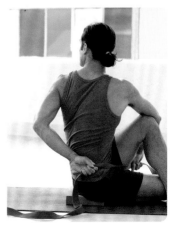

yoga *for health*

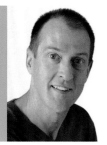

Yoga is a powerful tool for getting well and staying not just well, but better than well. What's its secret? Victoria Woodhall asks doctor and yoga teacher Timothy McCall MD

What are the health benefits of yoga?' In answer to this, their most frequently asked question, the International Association of Yoga Therapists (IAYT)[1] trawled through dozens of studies, papers and articles and drew up a comprehensive list of more than 60 physiological, psychological and biochemical benefits. These range from reduced blood pressure to the regulation of the endocrine, gastrointestinal and excretory functions, normalisation of weight, improved sleep, decreased anxiety and depression, better hand-eye coordination, improved memory and learning efficiency, increased white blood cell count, decreased LDL ('bad') cholesterol, and a general antistress and antioxidant effect, which is important in the prevention of degenerative diseases.

Yoga helps us when we are well by optimising the functioning of all the body's systems. When we are ill it can help manage symptoms such as fatigue, pain and low mood. It can even play a role in reversing disease. Dr Dean Ornish was the first to provide scientific proof that lifestyle changes including yoga and a low-fat diet could reverse heart disease, as well as lengthen telomeres (the ends of chromosomes that control ageing) and slow, stop or reverse the progression of early-stage prostate cancer.[2]

Yoga offers very simple tools to tackle stress, which can cause and worsen a whole host of health conditions. Among yoga's many therapeutic benefits are its effects on the mind. Bo Forbes, a clinical psychologist and yoga practitioner, is one teacher successfully using yoga programmes to help treat anxiety and depression.

But how is yoga such a powerful tool? Here, Dr Timothy McCall MD, author of *Yoga as Medicine: The Yogic Prescription for Health and Healing* and medical editor of *Yoga Journal*, shares his insights.

'AS SOMEONE WHO HAS BEEN A DOCTOR FOR almost 30 years, I can tell you that yoga is the most powerful overall system for promoting health and wellbeing I have ever seen. Why? Because we are working on immune function, the nervous system, the cardiovascular system, we are strengthening the muscles, improving flexibility, improving wellbeing, putting you in touch with your deeper purpose – what are you on the planet to do? Nothing in medicine deals with things like wellbeing, peacefulness, a sense of purpose and fulfilment – yet these are the things that matter most to us and have a huge impact on our health.

Yoga has a different view from Western medicine as to what constitutes health, and this may be partly why it is so effective. In medicine we take people who are symptomatic and try to make them less symptomatic. However, in yoga the absence of symptoms doesn't equate to health. Health extends far beyond not having a headache, knee pain or even curing cancer. It is about optimising the function of every system in your body.

When you bring a body into balance and improve posture and breathing, a lot of symptoms from back pain to insomnia will almost spontaneously get better.

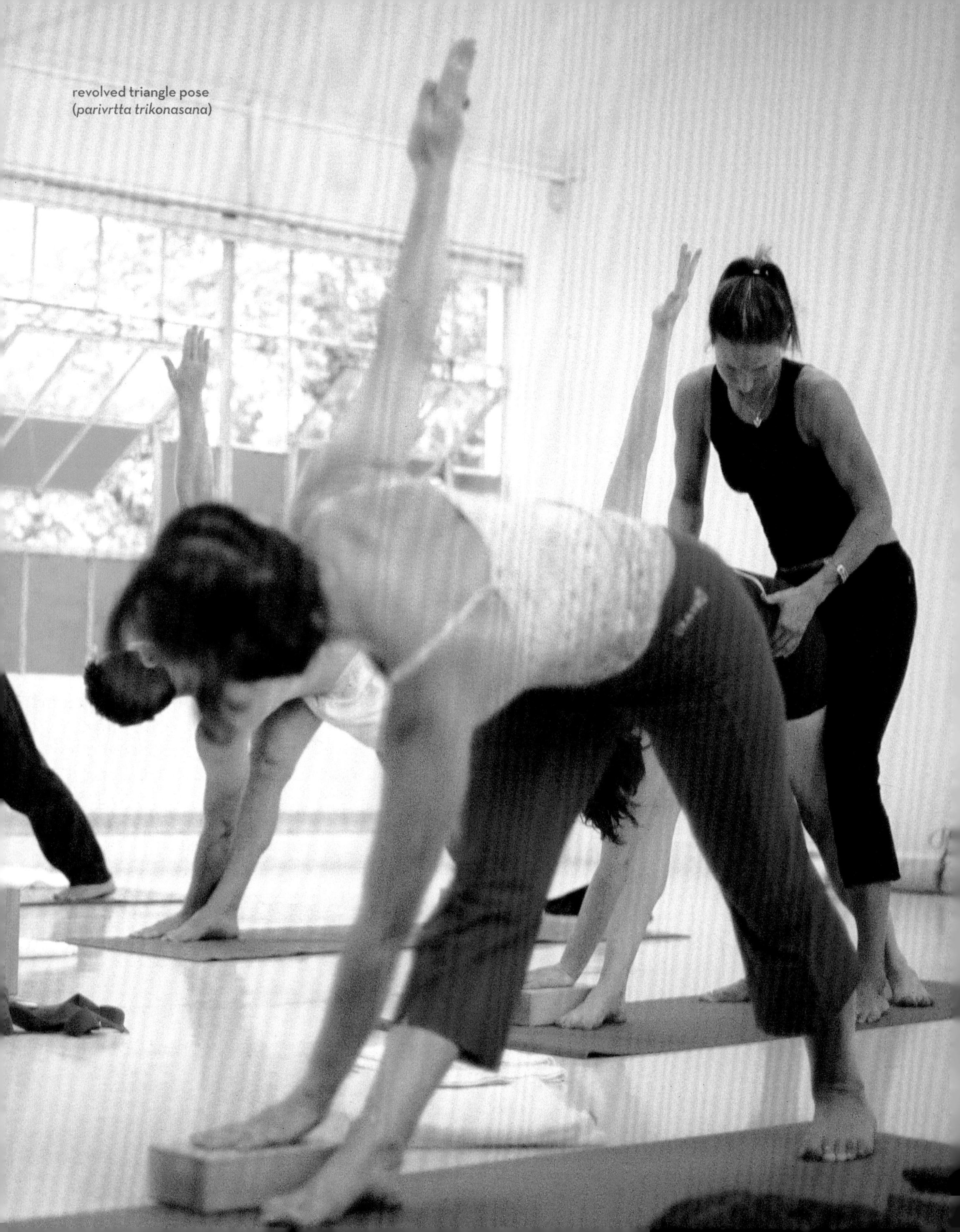

revolved triangle pose
(*parivrtta trikonasana*)

When you bring a body into balance and improve posture and breathing, a lot of symptoms from back pain to insomnia will almost spontaneously get better.

How does it work?

Yoga is a holistic practice that taps into dozens of systems that may have additive or even multiplicative effects. Stretching and lengthening the muscles calms the mind and can improve the breathing. Calming and strengthening the nervous system affects the mind. Cultivating peace of mind affects the nervous system, the immune system and the cardiovascular system.

Whether it's *asana*, *pranayama*, philosophy or meditation, yoga is a broad tool for tackling stress, which is a factor in some of the biggest health problems of our time. A lot of disease has a stress element to it – not just the things you might expect such as migraines, insomnia or irritable bowel syndrome, but also major diseases such as type 2 diabetes, depression, heart attacks and strokes, as well as autoimmune diseases such as MS and rheumatoid arthritis.

Something as simple as changing your posture can improve your breathing, which has all kinds of beneficial stress-reducing effects. But by and large, physicians know nothing about this. Doctors think about breathing only as a way of bringing more oxygen in to the body, not as a way of affecting your mental health or the state of your nervous system.

And yet we know as yogis that when we breathe differently it changes our nervous system and our anxiety levels, it affects our sleep, our mood, how well we interact with other people. Yoga takes into account a web of causation that is much more complex than the limited number of factors that most doctors consider.

Why is the breath so important?

It is perhaps the most important tool in yoga practice. The ancient yogis discovered that the breath, which is normally automatic, has profound effects on the nervous system if consciously controlled, with the potential either to increase activation or promote relaxation, depending on the practice.

The breath is our doorway into the whole autonomic nervous system (ANS) – the automatic functions (such as controlling heart rate, blood pressure, organ function and so on) that the body does by itself. Of all those automatic functions, the only one that almost everybody can take over voluntarily is the breath. When you change the breath, you change the ANS. In fact, some of the amazing feats that the ancient yogis developed, such as being able to sit naked outside in freezing temperatures, speeding or slowing down the heart or reducing their breathing to almost nothing, are due to the ability to control their nervous system. When you deepen and smooth out the breath, you are sending your ANS a signal of rest and relaxation instead of tension and potentially affecting all the internal organs, the blood, digestion, reproduction and so on. Slowing down the breath and making it more regular – with no major bumps or hiccups – begins to lessen feelings of stress within seconds. Yogic lore teaches that controlling the fluctuations of the breath helps calm the fluctuations of the mind.

All you need is yoga?

As preventative medicine, yoga is as close to one-stop shopping as you can find. While yoga by itself doesn't cure too much, there's almost nothing it can't help. Is yoga going to cure your cancer? No, but it might allow you to have more energy and fewer side-effects from treatment. The yogic approach does not say avoid all conventional medicine or don't ever take a drug or never have an operation. Instead we say that those are more tools.

In general, yoga helps us use fewer drugs and have fewer operations. If you have type 1 diabetes we are not going to say, 'Don't take your insulin, just do yoga' – that would be crazy. Use the drug, and complement it with yoga; or, the way I look at it, start with yoga and complement it with conventional medicine.

Yoga is strong medicine but it's slow medicine. If you want quick results or to feel better right away, you may need to consider conventional medical approaches. If you can be more patient, yoga can help you feel a little bit better right away, but the real deep effects come from continued practice over a long period.

How can it be used to heal?

Yoga wasn't originally invented to improve health or facilitate recovery from serious illness but as a spiritual path, to which disease was seen as an obstacle. However, there is a growing body of scientific evidence suggesting that yoga has serious therapeutic value. Studies have shown that it can benefit a wide variety of conditions from insomnia to attention deficit hyperactivity disorder (ADHD), multiple sclerosis, chronic pain, heart disease, depression and anxiety, rheumatoid arthritis, HIV/AIDS, alcoholism and drug withdrawal, to name but a few. When we use yoga therapeutically, we are not just addressing whatever physical problem the person is coming to us with, but also their overall situation, their stress levels, their posture, their breathing and, in as many ways as possible, are aiming to move them in a good direction.

One study I've been particularly impressed with is a two-year pilot into yoga's effectiveness for osteoporosis, published in 2009 by Loren Fishman MD, medical director of Manhattan Physical Medicine and Rehabilitation in New York.[3] He had people doing just ten minutes a day of *asana* and found dramatic improvements in bone mineral density. As impressive as that is, from a yogic perspective it's just the beginning. Yes, in yoga we are increasing bone mineral density but we are also making you less likely to fall and break a bone by improving your balance and by making you more mindful. And if you are about to fall, your core strength around your spine helps you right yourself. Then there's the fact that by learning to spread your toes and your metatarsal bones you actually widen your foot slightly, giving you a broader base for greater stability. When you have a wider foot, you are less likely to fall over; you are more stable. Yoga can also reduce the production of cortisol, the body's main stress hormone, which directly interferes with calcium deposition in the bone.

While health studies into yoga usually focus on one or a few specific effects – because that's the way we tend to measure success in medicine – they rarely tell the whole story, because there is often a raft of other benefits that may not be examined. So, looking back at the osteoporosis study, we learned that the patients'

bone mineral density improved but in all likelihood they also slept better and were happier as a result of their practice.

Is all yoga good for healing?

It's important to differentiate between yoga and yoga therapy. Take back pain, for example. There are now five randomised controlled studies that have found yoga to be effective (there are no randomised controlled studies that have shown that most back surgeries are effective). However, if you go to a general yoga class, it can make your back pain worse, or better, depending on how it's being taught and the nature of your back problem. If your back pain is caused by hyperextending (overarching) your lumbar (lower) spine and you go to a backbending class and are not careful, you are going to walk out of class in worse pain.

The average teacher in a health club isn't likely to know enough to teach therapeutic yoga well, especially not in a group setting. A yoga therapist, on the other hand, personalises the approach to what the individual needs. Yoga therapy is generally taught one-on-one or in small groups, often with the aid of props. With any injury or medical condition, unless it's minor, think carefully about going to a class, especially if you are not very experienced. Someone else is dictating the speed and the poses, which may not be what you need at that moment. Talk to the teacher, tell them your problem and ask them whether this is something they could manage in class. Err on the side of safety and listen to your body. If you start to feel a sharp pain, come out of the pose right away. Your body is giving you feedback. Unfortunately, in our achievement-oriented culture, many people feel like they need to push through. But in yoga it's 'pain, no gain'.

What's the pose for...?

A lot of people ask me, 'What's the pose for sinus problems' or 'What pose do I do if I have rheumatoid arthritis?' and the answer is always, 'It depends' – on the context of your whole life. How strong are you? How much time do you have to devote to yoga? What limitations do you have as a result of old injuries? What drugs are you taking? If you have a drug that makes you

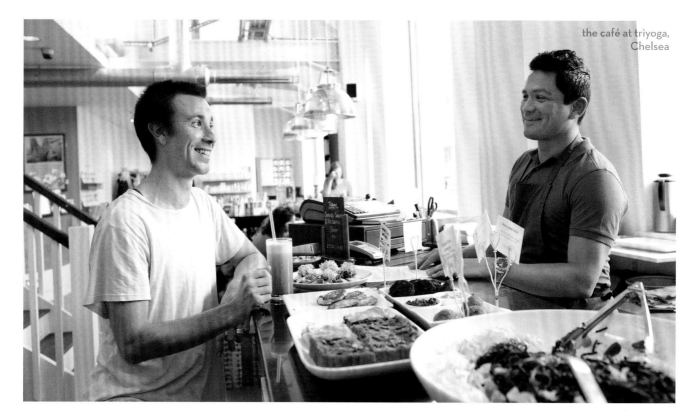

'I can tell you as a doctor, 'Don't eat that; it's bad
for you,' yet most of the time that advice goes in one
ear and out the other. But when it comes from
your own body, that's extremely motivating.'

dizzy, for example, we are going to think twice about putting you in a balancing pose.

When we use yoga therapeutically we are not just addressing whatever physical problem the person is coming to us with, but their overall situation. A yoga therapist will consider all these different things and come up with individual recommendations.

How often do I need to practise to experience health benefits?

You can feel the benefits from a single session, but if you want ongoing benefits that increase over time, you need to start a practice habit. The best way is to practise a small amount seven days a week. I would rather you did five minutes seven days a week than 20 minutes three times a week. By doing this you are creating what the ancient yogis called a *samskara* – a habit of action or a thought – making a mental groove that grows deeper the more you practise. By doing five minutes every day, you might find you want to do a bit more – six or ten minutes. Start with a little and let the practice itself convince you to do more. That's when the chance for profound change really begins.

How do I change old habits?

We all have neural pathways left by old habits and repetitive thoughts that live in our brain. How come, for example, someone who quit smoking 20 years ago can

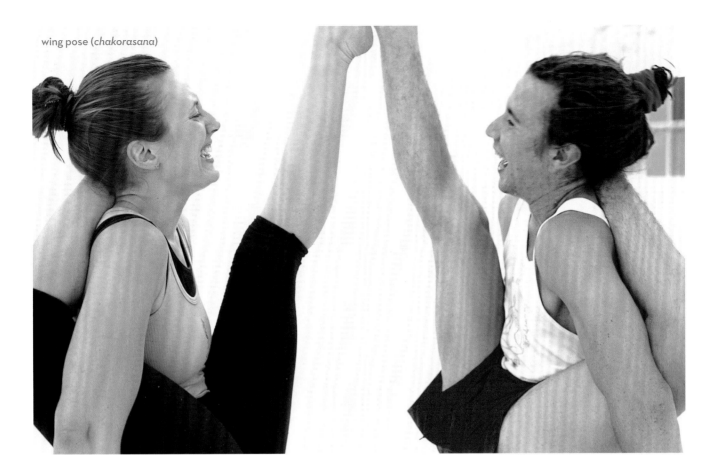
wing pose (*chakorasana*)

get fired from work, stop at a bar on the way home, have a few drinks, borrow a cigarette and the next day be smoking again? How did that happen? That old *samskara* was there, although somewhat attenuated through disuse. With yoga practice we create a new *samskara*, we repeat it until its gets stronger and gradually it starts to outcompete the old habits.

In creating *samskaras* we are forging new neural pathways. Until relatively recently, medical science believed that the brain was not capable of major change in adulthood. Now, with advances in understanding, scientists talk about neuroplasticity, meaning that the brain is capable of change. When you perform a new action or have a new thought, brain cells called neurons form new connections or synapses. The more you repeat it, the more synapses form and the stronger those neural pathways get. Neuroplasticity, I believe, is the neurological basis of the yogic idea of *samskaras* – and of Patanjali's recommendation of success in yoga, which is practice over a long period of time without

interruption. As yogis we can take advantage of neuroplasticity to change the structure of the brain.

Yoga makes you want to do what's good for you. How?

Yoga practice wakes up the ability to feel your own body. When you can feel the consequences of your behaviour, you start to make different decisions. Say, for example, you judge whether you can eat a particular food by whether you like how it tastes. When you can feel your own body, you might notice: 'Every time I eat that food I like the taste of, half an hour later I feel groggy and depressed.' You start to make the connection between the two and find yourself saying, 'I don't think I want to eat that food.'

I can tell you as a doctor, 'Don't eat that; it's bad for you,' yet most of the time that advice goes in one ear and out the other. But when it comes from your own body, that's extremely motivating. Part of what yoga does is it makes you want to do what's good for you.

stress – the Western world's biggest health issue

One of the chief factors undermining health and wellbeing in the modern world is an out-of-balance stress response. In a healthy stress response, the sympathetic nervous system (or SNS, an aspect of the autonomic nervous system) is temporarily activated when we perceive a threat – blood pressure goes up, blood sugar levels increase and our heart beats faster, bringing extra blood to the large muscles of the legs and arms for 'fight or flight', diverting it away from 'non-essential' functions such as digestion, the immune system and reproduction. When the threat passes, the parasympathetic nervous system (PNS) takes over and our body shifts into restorative mode – heart rate and stress hormone levels drop and blood is redirected to those non-essential functions.

Being nervous and on edge does have survival value. Even getting out of bed in the morning demands a surge in blood pressure that wouldn't happen without our built-in stress response. However, typical modern stressors – worries about relationships, jobs, money, security – tend not to be resolved as quickly as the physical threats our ancestors faced, so our stress response system stays activated or is repeatedly reactivated. When our stress response is out of balance in this way, the system that was designed to protect us from danger can do the opposite and cause disease.

What's more, elevated levels of the stress hormone cortisol have been linked to increased blood sugar levels, high blood pressure, stress-related overeating and laying-down of unhealthy abdominal fat, which increases the risk of the major killers type 2 diabetes and heart disease. Yoga gives us powerful tools to lower activity in the SNS and increase activity in the PNS. Stress is often fuelled by worried thoughts. Yoga teaches you to stop your mind working against you – in the words of Patanjali, by 'slowing the fluctuations of the mind'. Over time yoga helps us realise that much of what we get upset about is not that important – and that realisation may be the best stress reduction method of all.
– Timothy McCall MD

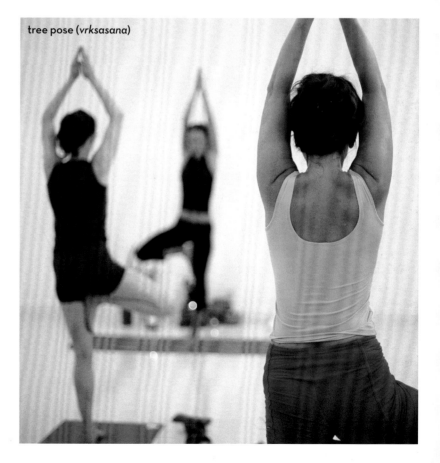

tree pose (*vrksasana*)

yoga for men

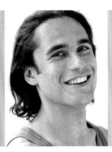

If 30 million people in the world do yoga, why is it mostly women who make up the numbers? Victoria Woodhall asks Jeff Phenix, 'What's holding men back?'

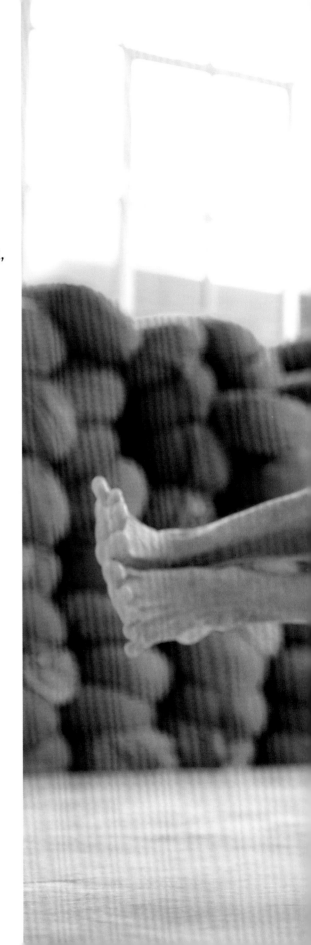

If we look at who comes through the door at triyoga, women outnumber men by about four to one, if not more. In teacher-training groups the numbers of men can sometimes be as low as one in 15. Despite the fact that yoga comes from a strong male lineage and that many of the poses that originated in India were essentially designed for male bodies (which some women even now complain about – think of trying a shoulder stand with a GG chest!), in the West yoga can often be seen as something of a closed door for men. It doesn't help that magazine articles tend to be illustrated with a pretty size-eight model sitting serenely in lotus or striking a tree pose against the sunset. Where's the man in baggy shorts with the paunch, more interested in improving his bad back than his karma? If you are a man reading this, who has never done yoga before, you probably think it's something you should do, but somewhere there may be a resistance that stops you setting foot in a class (many male practitioners tell us they started yoga from a book).

One physiotherapist, a three-times-a-week tennis player in his thirties, told us that while he would recommend yoga as a remedial exercise for someone who had an injury, he wouldn't consider taking it up himself. He would miss his 'workout' and the competitive side of tennis where he could measure his performance by his scores.

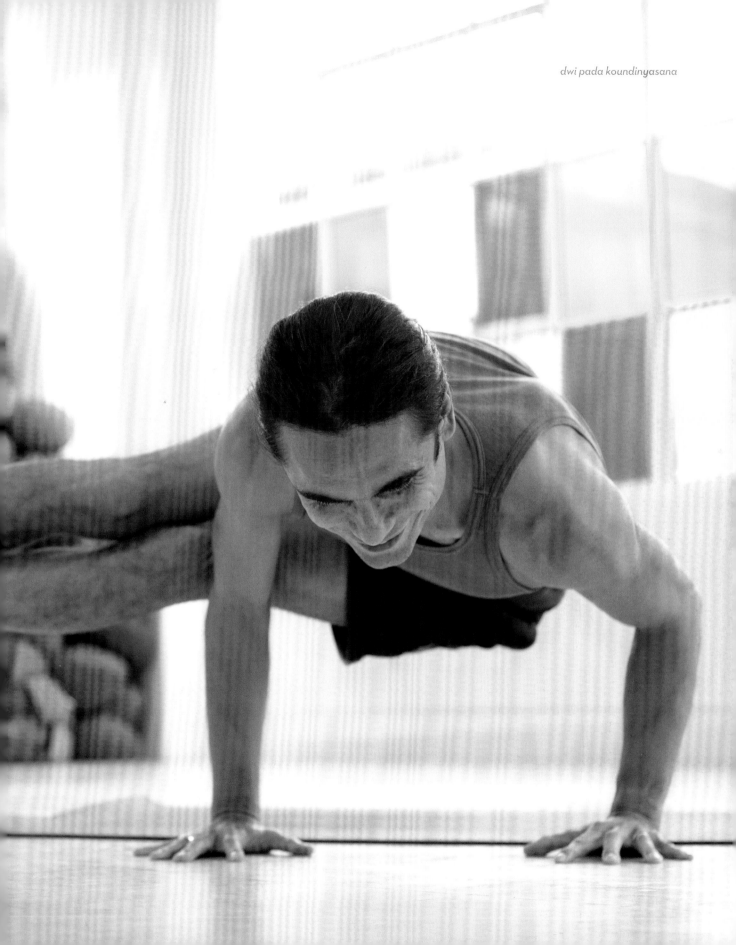

dwi pada koundinyasana

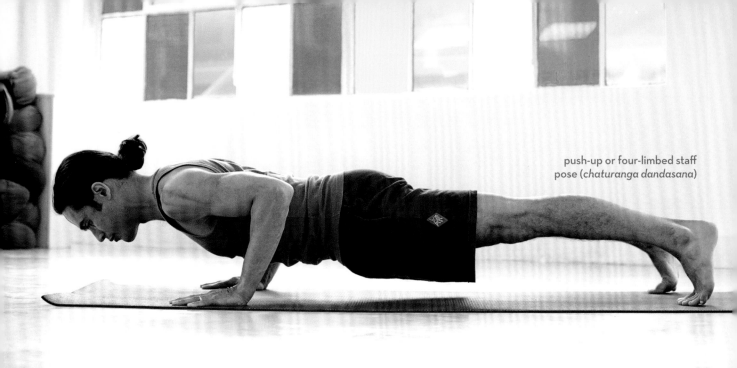

push-up or four-limbed staff pose (*chaturanga dandasana*)

One way of looking at yoga as a competitive sportsman, is as a discipline to help keep you injury free. In 20 years from now when other people's bones are starting to creak and old injuries start to nag, you are more likely still to be playing. If you like to sweat and to measure your performance in numbers, try vinyasa flow, or Ashtanga – in which there are six sequences of ever-increasing difficulty.

Yoga is a powerful tool for so many things – stress relief, improved sporting performance, better focus, fuller range of movement as well as general health – and there's no good reason for anyone, male or female, to miss out. It sharpens the mind-body connection and trains you to be in the present, really to be aware of what's going on around you, to stay calm when life becomes challenging. People who do yoga alongside their sport report that they are better able to see advantages – such as a space opening up on the pitch or court. Increasingly, top athletes from across a range of sporting disciplines, as well as entrepreneurs, business leaders and politicians, are turning to yoga because it helps their performance without blunting their competitive nature.

Having a clear, calm mind and a healthy body gives you the edge, whether that's in sport, business or life generally. Happily, more men are starting to realise this.

FOUR YOGA MYTHS UNRAVELLED

MYTH 1: It's for girls

If you are a man, yoga might not feel like a natural fit for you – all that stretching can seem challenging even if you are very fit and do a lot of sport. Women are by and large more flexible than men and are more likely to choose yoga as their main fitness activity; hence its 'female' image. Men tend to prefer their 'weekend warrior' pursuits.

Men can find yoga a challenge not only physically, but mentally too, says Jeff. 'It can be tough when you are surrounded by women who all seem to be better at it than you. It takes time and a bit of humility to break through that mental resistance.

'I teach a group of women golfers who say they have fewer aches and pains, that they feel better in their bodies and that their game has improved. But when they tried to persuade their men to come along, the husbands couldn't get past the teasing from their peers. The notion that yoga is somehow effeminate can terrify men. They think it's a bit balletic, a bit tree-huggy, that they'll look silly or not get anything useful out of it.

'Luckily, with top sportsmen and businessmen now "coming out" about their yoga practice, this perception is gradually changing.'

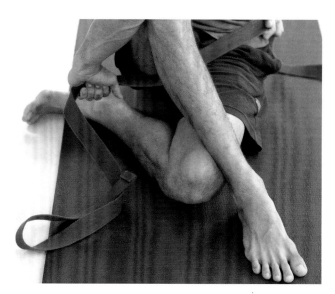

Luckily, with top sportsmen and businessmen now 'coming out' about their yoga practice, perceptions are gradually changing.

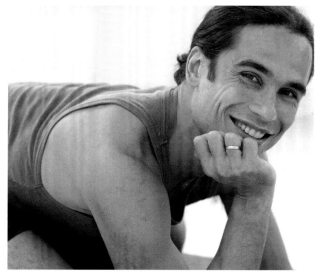

MYTH 2: It's not a proper workout

'The reason why everybody likes yoga is that it isn't very hard.' So said a celebrity fitness trainer recently in a UK national newspaper. This is just the sort of unhelpful comment that puts many people off – especially men. 'Many men don't realise that there are dozens of styles of yoga and that they can find one that allows them to work as hard as they like,' says Jeff. Yoga teacher Baron Baptiste, who acted as a performance coach to the Philadelphia Eagles football team, reports that in his experience men tend to get hooked into stronger styles because they 'connect with the power of the practice'.[1]

'Even Olympic athletes (with the possible exception of gymnasts) would find certain types of yoga, such as Ashtanga, a challenge,' says Jeff.

You are not going to bulk up like a bodybuilder by doing yoga, nor are you going to get marathon-fit. But you will work your cardiovascular system and develop longer, leaner, more balanced muscles that will not only support whatever sport you play, but are also useful in other areas of your life – twisting around to reverse the car, swinging a golf club; lifting your child up without doing your back in; reaching up to the top of the wardrobe to get a suitcase. This 'real life' fitness becomes more important as we age. Gyms are now recognising this and buzzwords such as 'evolutionary

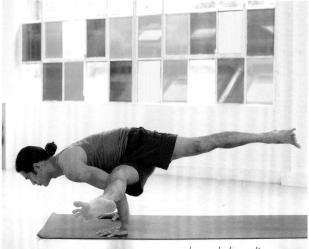

eka pada koundinyasana

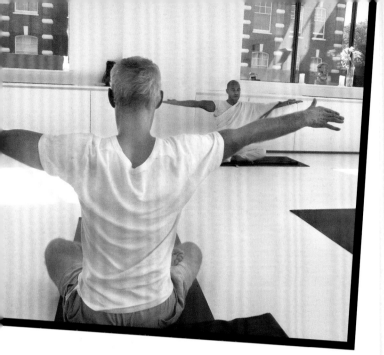

movement' and 'functional fitness' are creeping in, ushering out the 1980s six-pack aesthetic and bulky, overtrained muscles. The 'evolutionary' or 'primal' approach takes the body through all the movements it was designed to do.

Yoga has known this all along – we need to access a full range of motion to stay healthy and strong and to use all muscles in balance.

MYTH 3: I'm not bendy enough

Flexibility is not a requirement for yoga but it comes with practice. Everyone works non-competitively at their own 'edge'.

'Yoga is extremely beneficial for men, because it addresses our typical problem areas – tight shoulders, hips, hamstrings and quads plus legs that are weak relative to upper body strength, and a weak core,' says Jeff. 'All of these can contribute to low back pain, which men also frequently report. In time your body will balance out. The muscles are then better able to support one another, spreading the work more evenly and efficiently.' On a physical level, yoga is about balancing strength with flexibility.

In the meantime there are ways out of every tight spot with simple adjustments, props and an attitude of 'less is sometimes more'.

Getting out of a tight spot by Jeff Phenix

Tight shoulders: A bulky upper body can make common poses such as downward facing dog tricky. Tightness in the biceps means it may be hard for you to straighten the arms, reducing stability in the shoulders. A bulky upper body might also make binding in a twist more tricky.
Try this: In downward facing dog **(a)**, take the hands slightly wider apart with index fingers pointing straight ahead. In bound twist **(b)**, use a strap to bridge the gap between the hands.

Tight hamstrings: If the backs of your legs are tight, trying to touch your toes when bending forward or to straighten the legs in downward facing dog may overwork the back, causing it to hunch (see forward-bending instructions in the practice section, page 136).
Try this: In seated forward bends **(c)**, use a belt to bridge the gap between your hands and feet or **(d)** sit on blocks to help elevate the hips and lengthen the spine. In standing forward bends, place your hands on blocks. Make sure you bend at the hips, not the lower back. In downward facing dog **(e)**, keep the back straight but bend the knees.

Tight hips: If your knees are higher than your hips when you sit cross-legged, it means that the thighs and hips are too tight to allow the knees to lower. These muscles are easily shortened if you spend a lot of time sitting on a chair or driving or doing sports. Your pelvis may also tilt backwards, causing you to slump, putting strain on your back.
Try this: Sit on the edge of a block **(f)** – or a pile of blocks – to raise your seat higher. Your knees should lower and you should feel your spine growing taller.

Tight quads (thighs): These can restrict your backbends and make postures such as pigeon and hero pose **(g)**, challenging.
Try this: Use extra support under your buttocks to bring the floor to you.

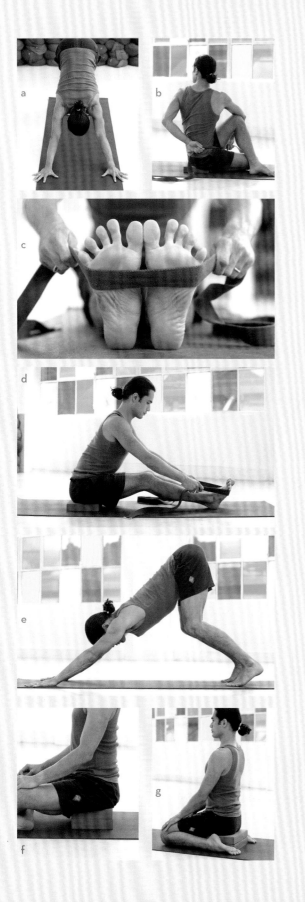

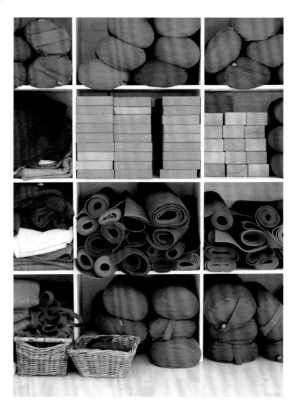

A WORD ON PROPS

Belts and foam blocks allow you to get the full benefits of a difficult pose by taking your body where it won't yet go by itself. Props aren't cheating – in fact, in the Iyengar method, some poses exist only with props.

'Props keep the lines of energy in your body clearer, which is unlikely to happen if you muscle into a pose through brute strength,' says Jeff. 'If you are screwing up your eyes or puffing and panting, you are overworking – it's a common male trait. Our practical "doing" mindset says, "It's a workout, therefore I should be Working Out." In class, it's always the men sweating buckets. Pushing too hard leads to tightening, which can restrict the flow of breath and energy. It took time for me to learn to work with the breath rather than the feeling of needing to achieve. Once you learn to work with subtlety and refinement you realise that sometimes you can go further by doing less.'

In yoga a natural competitiveness can also be turned inwards as a means of becoming better in yourself.

MYTH 4: It will make me less competitive

Will all that yoga blunt your edges and ambition? The growing number of figures in big business who use yoga to help them stay at the top of their game suggests that this can't be true. The improved mental clarity, focus and ability to manage stress gained through yoga are important skills in a world swamped by emails, tweets and texts, and defined by economic uncertainty. In yoga, a natural competitiveness can also be turned inwards as a means of becoming better in yourself.

Early adopters include Guy Hands, multi-millionaire chairman of private equity company Terra Firma, who does yoga before work.[2] Bill Gross, America's 'bond king', says he has some of his most inspired ideas while standing on his head and that after practice 'a light bulb turns on and I'm on to something'.[3] Russell Simmons, multimillionaire founder of Def Jam Records and Phat Farm clothing, is a long-time Jivamukti yoga devotee and has written a book *Super Rich* based on yogic principles.

Yoga can even look good on your CV. One head of human resources at a corporate law firm reportedly recommended the candidate who did yoga over their equally qualified rival.[4]

In the world of sport, it's becoming increasingly common to hear of yoga being part of an elite training regime – fans include UK football Premiership stars Roy Keane and Ryan Giggs. (Giggs, still playing in his late 30s, attributes his career longevity to yoga[5] – and he even released a yoga-based fitness DVD.) Entire teams such as Tottenham Hotspur and Arsenal, the 2011 Welsh rugby World Cup squad, and the Philadelphia Eagles football team all do yoga. In tennis, Andy Murray and Rafael Nadal both practise regularly.

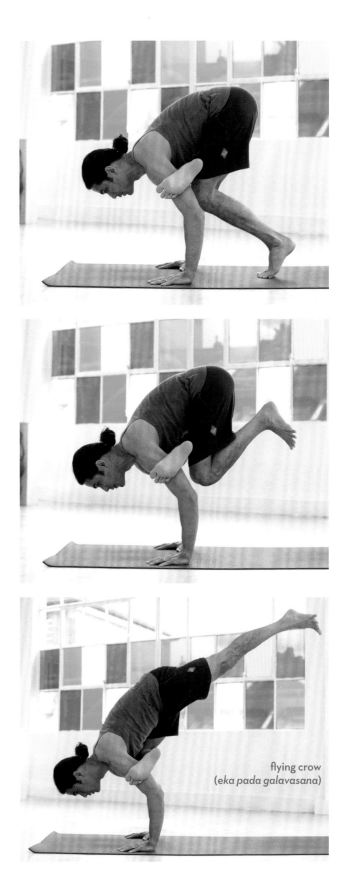

flying crow
(*eka pada galavasana*)

Five-and-a-half reasons for men to do yoga:

1. Improved physical and mental performance

Yoga trains all muscle groups to work together, sharing the load. This means that some are less likely to become tired or injured through overwork, and to become weak or even switch off through underuse.

Whatever physical activity you do in daily life, from sport to pushing your child on a swing, you will do more effectively. Improved concentration and focus help with mental performance and decision-making off the mat too.

2. Staying youthful

Yoga puts the body through its full range of motion, twisting, reaching, stretching, moving from sitting on the floor to standing. As we get older we can retain that range of movement in the face of the natural shrinking of the muscles over time. Yoga increases energy and regular practice often results in making healthier choices over diet, handling stress, and getting enough sleep – all things that make us look and feel young. 'Yogis tend to be more flexible, stronger, more energetic, thinner and more youthful than people who don't do yoga,' says Dr Timothy McCall.[6]

3. Dealing better with stress

Yoga helps us relax. Breathing more slowly and deeply oxygenates the blood and calms the mind, grounding us in the face of stress. Certain types of yoga, such as restorative yoga, focus particularly on activating the parasympathetic nervous system (our relaxation response) taking us out of 'fight or flight' mode and reducing stress hormones.

4. Better concentration and focus

Yoga and meditation develop mental clarity, training the ability to connect with what's going on in the present moment and to screen out distractions.

5. Relieving back pain

Several studies show that yoga can be effective for back pain, a common complaint for men. 'It's where medicine does the poorest job and yoga does the best,' says Dr Timothy McCall.[7]

5½. Getting a better beach body

You know you care – just a little bit. Yoga trains long, lean, balanced muscles that look great in swimming trunks. What's not to like?

Whatever physical activity you do in daily life, from sport to pushing your child on a swing, you will do more effectively

yoga for women

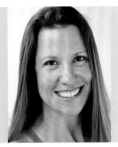

Men and women both share the same physical blueprint for healthy and harmonious alignment. However, there are fundamental physical differences between the sexes (not just the obvious!) and an appreciation of these may help you practise with more sensitivity

BY AYALA GILL

As women, we are constantly adapting physically and emotionally to our changing bodies and roles. As we change – not only month to month, but through adolescence, pregnancy, motherhood and beyond – our yoga practice can change to support us.

For me, this is a great blessing because it compels me to be more sensitive. The more I listen to myself in my yoga practice and respond to what I actually need (rather than what I want, or think I need), the better it supports me.

A deep connection to what is going on in the moment – whether we like that experience or not – can lead us to a yoga practice that is authentic and transformative. Authentic because we are responding in a genuine, honest way to ourselves rather than being ruled by our ego or our fears; and transformative because we can only grow when we begin where we are right now, rather than where we think we should be.

HOW IS A WOMAN'S BODY DIFFERENT?

1. Lower centre of gravity

Broader hips mean that a woman's centre of gravity is generally in her pelvis, whereas a man's is in his broader chest. This affects the way we do poses such as arm balances (such as crow, handstand) and push-up **(a)**, (*chaturanga dandasana*) because here our centre of gravity is further from our foundation – in this case our hands. Because our weight feels very heavy in our arms, we might skip these poses, mistakenly assuming that lack of arm strength is the sole issue.

Try this: Work the legs more strongly (to feel this action in *chaturanga* try squeezing a block between the thighs as shown). Doing this redistributes the weight of our pelvis and we are better able to access the exhilaration that these poses offer.

2. Broader hips

A man's thigh bones are set close together and travel more directly up to the pelvis than a woman's, which are set wider apart and turn more of a corner at the hip socket.

The result is that we can struggle to get the correct actions of the inner legs in front-facing poses, such as intense side stretch, *parsvottanasana* **(see b, over)** and warrior 1, and in seated forward bends if we do them with the classical alignment of feet together.

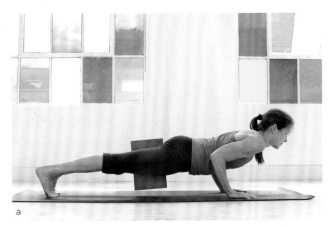

a

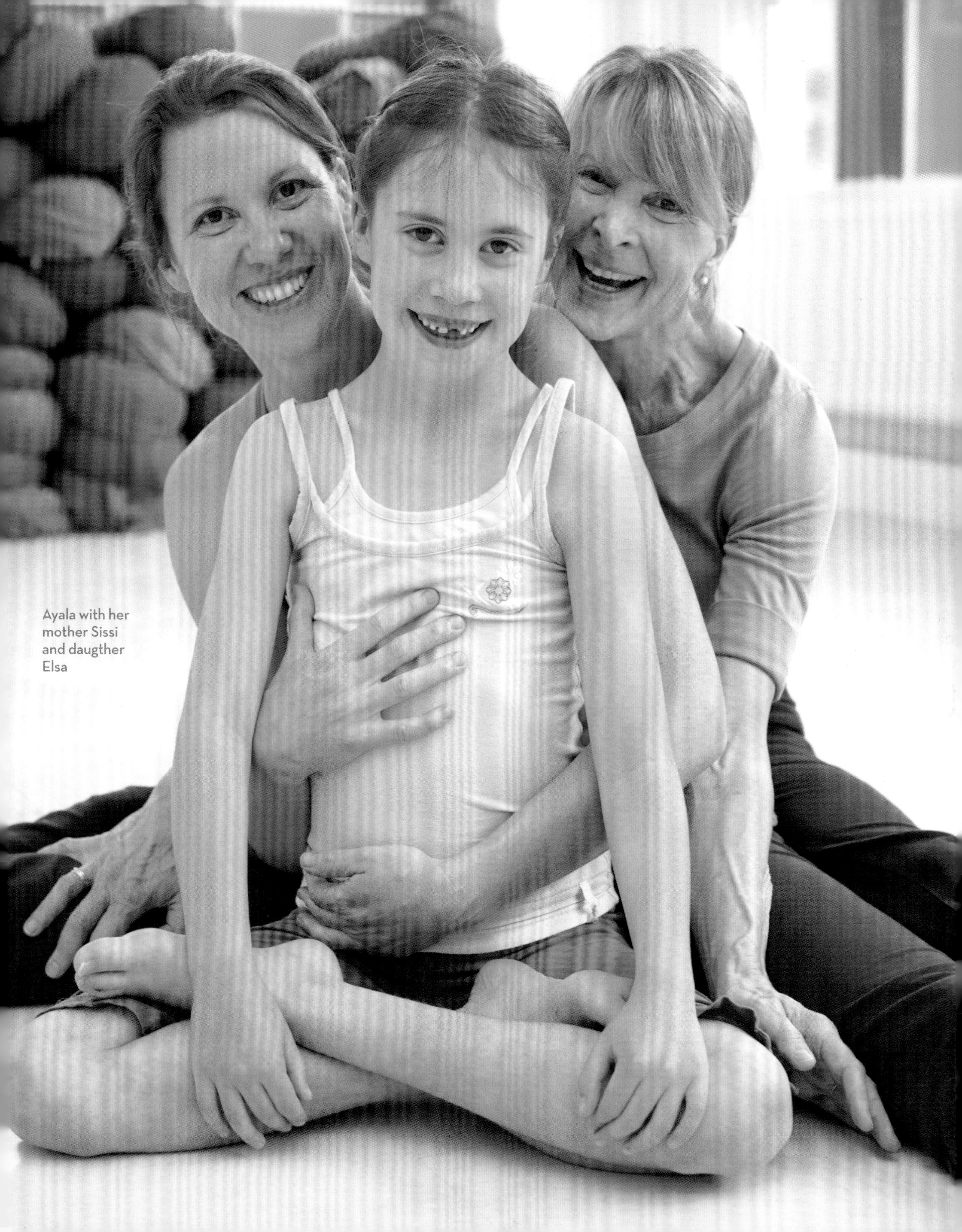

Ayala with her
mother Sissi
and daugther
Elsa

Try this: Wider stance – place your feet hip-width apart in these poses to make the correct actions of the inner legs more accessible (inner legs lifting up, inner groins moving backwards and apart). Then lengthen your tailbone down and firm the outer hips. This creates a harmonious alignment of the legs, pelvis and spine, which in turn creates lightness and lift in the inner body.

3. Less muscular bulk

This is a mixed blessing. On the one hand we have a greater range of movement because we are not restricted by tightness or muscular bulk, but on the other hand we can't rely on natural stiffness to keep our joints stable. On top of this, hormonal changes during menstruation, pregnancy and breast-feeding soften the ligament support around our joints and, as we age, our muscles tend to move away from our bones.

Try this: Engage the muscles so that they come close to the bones and the arms and legs draw towards the midline. This integrates and stabilises the muscles and joints, from which we can then extend outwards safely,

while expanding our inner body effortlessly.

4. Sacroiliac joint

Women are eight to ten times more likely to suffer from sacroiliac pain than men. The sacroiliac joint **(c)**, which consists of a series of ligaments joining the sacrum (the flat upside-down triangle-shaped bone at the base of the spine) to the pelvis, is not designed for a large range of movement since its major function is stability. A woman's wider hips mean that everyday activities such as walking create more movement in this joint than in men. Our wider pelvis also means that the joint is shallower, so a smaller part of the sacrum is able to attach to the pelvis. Add to this the hormonal softening of ligaments at certain times of the month and we have an area that is always going to be vulnerable in women. Yoga can help strengthen the supporting muscles, and correct alignment can prevent sacroiliac pain occuring in the first place.

Try this: Simple backbends – locust **(d)**, cobra and bow pose can strengthen the supporting muscles as long as

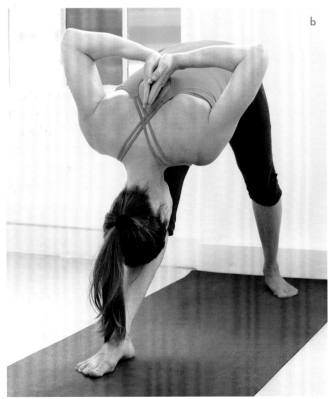

b

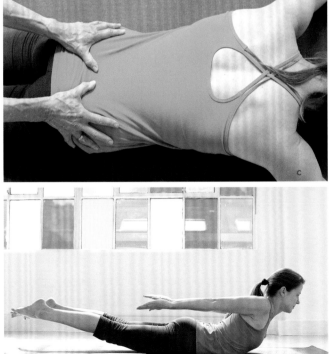

d

they are practised correctly (with thighs spiralling inwards, buttock muscles firm and tailbone lengthening away from the sacrum) so that the area stays broad.

Take care also in twists and forward bends. We may think of these as primarily a movement of the spine, but if we leave the pelvis behind it's the sacroiliac joint nestling between them that takes the strain. The answer once again lies in working the legs correctly, so that with the thighs fixed we can initiate forward bending or twisting from the pelvis and so protect the sacroiliac joint.

5. The reproductive organs

The way we hold our belly influences how effectively our reproductive and digestive organs function. In our culture, many women aspire to a flat stomach and may have been pulling in their abdominal muscles for most of their adult lives. It's not just body consciousness that can cause a perpetually gripped abdomen; stress, fear and anxiety can also often manifest in this way. Hardening the diaphragm and belly – and the throat too – causes us to feel less and is often an automatic response when we feel overwhelmed.

We may not even realise how 'gripped' we are in the belly since many of us feel disconnected from this area. This may be because of previous trauma, or simply because of living in a headstrong culture in which our body can feel like another (little-visited) planet!

All of this reduces circulation to these vital organs, and can lead to fertility, menstrual and digestive issues. To function properly, our digestive and reproductive organs need to be elongated and soft **(e)**, rather than constricted or congested, and the supporting muscles long and strong rather than permanently cramped. Yoga teaches us how to tone and align the body for this to happen.

Try this: 1) Neutral pelvis – standing so that the pelvis is neutral, not tilted forwards or back, holds organs in their proper place. The abdominal muscles can then do their real job of helping us to breathe, aligning the pelvis, containing the organs and assisting with stability and movement of the torso.

2) Breathe into the belly. On a psychological level,

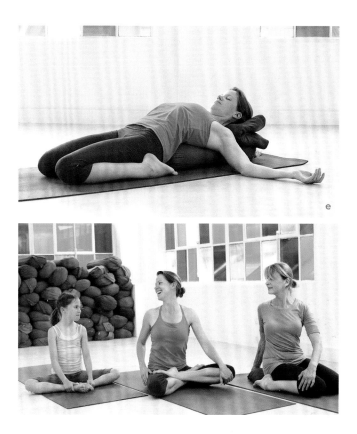

e

yoga encourages us to be open to what we are feeling, both good and bad. The more we do this, the less our need to 'keep it all in', packed away in tight, hard muscles, and the more we learn to welcome (or at least acknowledge) the experiences that come our way. In directing our attention to the belly through breathing, stretching and strengthening, we can begin to reacquaint ourselves with this area. This is the first step on a long journey of self-acceptance, which culminates in letting go of the distorted image of ourselves we may have been holding on to, and celebrating the person we are.

BODY IMAGE AND EATING DISORDERS

Psychological and emotional factors are complex in relation to compulsive eating disorders: triggers can range from controlling food to gain a sense of control in a world that increasingly fails to make sense, to using food to block out overwhelming emotions and pain.

A 2004 study published in the *Psychology of Women Quarterly*[1] found that women who practised yoga had a healthier attitude towards their bodies and fewer disordered eating behaviours than those who did aerobic exercise.

A well-rounded yoga practice can support women with eating disorders in many ways. Standing poses help with feeling strong and grounded, teaching you to find your own power and presence in the world. Backbends, such as locust, bow and *urdhva dhanurasana* (pictured below), open up the chest and increase vitality and capacity to feel loving, towards yourself as well as others. Inversions are emotionally balancing and stabilising.

It is important, however, that you are honest with yourself and are not using your practice to fuel your compulsion further: are you drawn to a rigorous practice as a means to burn more calories? If you are attracted to a dynamic practice, instead of using it as another tool for control, can you learn to apply curiosity and loving attention to your body in the more physically demanding poses?

When your attention is harnessed in a loving way towards exploring strength, flexibility and balance, there may no longer be room for your compulsive inner critic to be at the forefront. Over time you may find the courage to apply this same attention to whatever thoughts and feelings reveal themselves in your final relaxation (*savasana*). Because the focus of a yoga practice is on feeling your body from the inside, rather than on appearance, you begin to find security in a new feeling of wholeness and slowly build courage to meet painful parts of yourself.

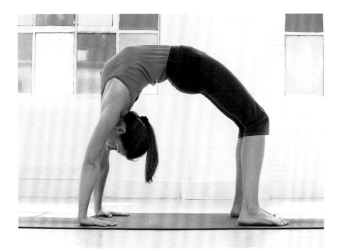

menstrual practice – the basics

1. Create space. Choose poses which bring gentle elongation and breadth to the reproductive organs, liver and kidneys. These include forward bends, gentle backbends, seated and supine poses **(a)**, all of which should be well supported by props so that the front and back of the body remain long and broad. For a detailed description of menstrual practices, see Lois Steinberg's *Geeta S. Iyengar's Guide to a Woman's Yoga Practice*, volume 1, or Linda Sparrowe and Patricia Walden's *The Woman's Book of Yoga and Health*.

2. Head off headaches. If your head is feeling heavy due to tension, begin your practice with a child's pose (*balasana*), cross-legged forward bend (*adho mukha svastikasana*) or standing forward bend (*uttanasana*) **(b)**, all with your head resting on a chair or bolsters.

3. Relieve pain. If you are having heavy bleeding or a painful period, try half moon pose (*ardha chandrasana*) **(c)** against the wall to make space in the pelvis and abdomen. According to Geeta Iyengar, this pose also has a drying effect on the uterus.

4. Energise hard-working liver and kidneys. Try Yin yoga poses emphasising the kidney meridian (butterfly pose **(d)**, seal pose) and liver meridian (shoelace pose **(e)**, dragonfly pose). According to Chinese medicine, the kidney *chi* (energy) supports our reproductive health, whilst the liver *chi* helps to balance our emotions. For a detailed description of these poses, see *Insight Yoga* by Sarah Powers.

5. Check in with yourself. I use these quiet menstrual poses to notice whether I've been practising from my ego or whether I have been giving myself what I really need to nourish my body and spirit. Many women begin a practice of attuning with themselves during their monthly cycle, and in time begin to apply this sensitive listening to each practice, each day.

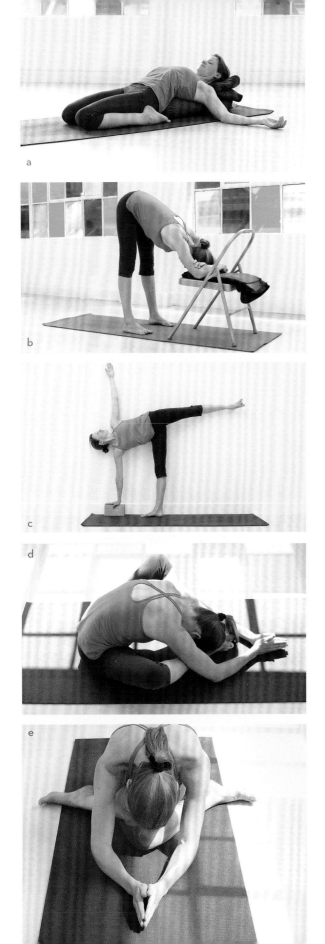

a

b

c

d

e

PRACTISING DURING YOUR PERIOD

I like the term 'moon cycle', which is increasingly being used in yoga to describe our period, because the way we feel it sometimes mirrors the moon's waxing and waning (the word 'menstruation' is also related to the word 'moon'). We move from feeling light, outgoing and creative to becoming darker, more reflective and withdrawn. During our period, the body cleans out the uterus and gathers the general hormonal detritus that has built up during the month and moves it out with the menstrual blood. This is a time when the liver and kidneys, as organs of detoxification, have to work hard.

If we ignore what our body is trying to do and plough on with our regular active practice, we risk interfering with this natural process of renewal. But if we don't practise at all during our period, we will miss out on the benefits of yoga – namely supporting the organs so they can do their job well, which will minimise discomfort and irregularities in our cycle.

Energetically, the downward energy of *apana vayu* is increased (see page 167). Crucially for menstruation, this helps us with elimination. During this time I want to support this releasing of energy, so I do not practise inversions. Inversions also pull your uterus towards your waist, which can cause the broad ligaments around it to overstretch.

What's more, inversions require the legs to be very active to support the spine. During menstruation the legs should not be overexerted as they relate to the earth and fire elements which both need to be pacified for a healthy hormonal balance at this time, according to women's yoga expert Geeta Iyengar.[2] For this reason she advises avoiding strenuous standing poses, and doing those that are recommended with the support of the wall.

Finally, I also avoid all poses which harden or strongly twist the abdomen, such as push-up (*chaturanga dandasana*), boat pose (*navasana*) and half lord of the fishes pose (*ardha matsyendrasana*). Your period is not the time to push forward in your practice, but to make space in your body and direct your breath downwards to wherever you feel hardness or cramping.

FERTILITY – HOW YOGA CAN SUPPORT YOU

Yoga has an important role in supporting fertility. In yoga, infertility implies an imbalance in the *svadhisthana* chakra: the energy centre located between the navel and pubic bone that controls the reproductive organs. Having a chronically 'gripped' abdomen diminishes the energy circulating in this area. The restorative or Yin practices suggested for menstruation are also beneficial for improving fertility since they support the reproductive system. When you are not menstruating, a regular inversion practice is also essential to maintain hormonal balance (inversions nourish the pituitary, pineal and thyroid glands). Supported inversions, such as legs-up-the-wall pose (*viparita karani*), and shoulder stand with a chair (*salamba sarvangasana*, right) allow you to stay longer in the poses and receive more benefit.

Balancing masculine and feminine

From a traditional Chinese medical perspective, we can also address infertility by considering where there is an imbalance between the masculine and feminine aspects of ourselves. The Taoist principles of *yin* and *yang* suggest that *yin* embodies the feminine and *yang* the masculine. When these two elements are out of balance, there is disease in the body. It has been well documented, for example, that some women who overemphasise *yang* activities (heating, upward moving and dynamic, such as strong athletic training, or a strong dynamic yoga practice) can find their menstrual cycle is disrupted or stops altogether. The way a woman's body responds to such activities will depend on her individual constitution.

If we understand our physical/emotional/mental make-up more clearly (with the support of an Ayurvedic practitioner or traditional Chinese doctor, for instance) we can choose a yoga practice that brings genuine balance. But ultimately the style of yoga you practise perhaps matters less than your capacity to bring the qualities you are looking to cultivate with you on to the mat. For fertility, our primary aims are to bring space and vitality to the lower belly, and to reduce our levels of stress.

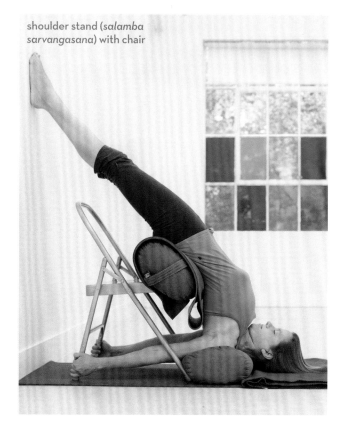

shoulder stand (*salamba sarvangasana*) with chair

Fertility and stress

Stress is one of the main enemies of fertility. The stress hormone adrenaline constricts blood vessels, possibly including those in the uterus, thus interfering with conception. Stress hormones also wreak havoc with the fertility hormones.

As if this weren't enough, after the age of 35 we start to produce less of these sex hormones, while our bodies also become less able to deal with stress hormones. So, according to Ayurvedic practitioner Dr Claudia Welch, we have a scenario where the impact of stress is more at the same time as our natural capacity to conceive is lessening.[3]

Even with all this evidence in favour of slowing down, it can be daunting to think what would happen if we stepped out of our stressful circumstances. Indeed, the stress of trying to conceive is itself enormous. A yoga practice can help us to shift our focus from a need to achieve towards being healthy and awake in this moment. We relax some grip on our desire to conceive, and focus instead on revitalising our body and opening our hearts to the possibility of conception.

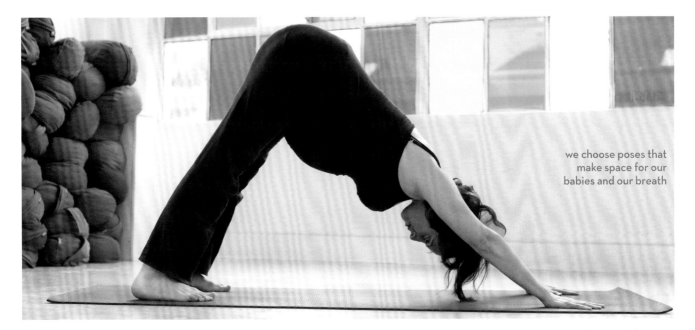

we choose poses that
make space for our
babies and our breath

PREGNANCY AND BIRTH

Pregnancy is a wonderful time to practise yoga. Because we are practising for our babies as well as ourselves, we have a greater responsibility than at other times. But we also have greater potential for benefit. On a physical level, we choose poses that make space for our babies as well as our breath. Our lungs, diaphragm and digestive organs all become compressed as our babies grow, so we learn how to lengthen the spine and broaden the diaphragm to maximise the space in the inner body. Hormones also cause joints to become more mobile, so we learn how to use our muscles to stabilise the joints and support our babies.

On an emotional and psychological level, our yoga practice is an opportunity to connect with our babies and listen to how we are really feeling. It is a time when all our tendencies – physical, emotional and mental – seem to become magnified, but at the same time our attention naturally moves towards our babies, leaving us more introverted and reflective. So while a lot of issues might arise during pregnancy, there is often a greater willingness to look closely at them. I see many women grow in strength and conviction during pregnancy: it is a time when we sift out what truly matters from what is simply demanding on our time. Sometimes women feel guilty if they are not enjoying

their pregnancy. One of the wonderful aspects of yoga philosophy is that instead of implying that pregnancy should be a blissful experience, we are simply guided towards connecting with ourselves, and offering the same love to ourselves that we are beginning to feel for our baby. As a result, we can start to feel some ease and spaciousness even in the midst of turmoil. Yoga explores ways to invite in everything that we are experiencing, including uncomfortable sensations or feelings of fear. As we allow these experiences to simply rest in loving attention, we wake up to the full technicolour spectrum of our lives.

When we discover that we are able to use these tools to remain present during the enormous challenge of giving birth, it can be profoundly empowering. I like to encourage women to aspire to a 'connected' birth above all. If our intention is to stay open to the experience of birth, with a willingness to listen to the signals from our body and baby without resistance, the chances of a natural delivery increase. When we are surrounded by others who are able to support this intention, it becomes still more powerful. If medical intervention is then genuinely needed, we can welcome it without feeling any sense of failure or disappointment. As women, we can endure incredible difficulty and challenge as long as we are both connected to that experience and supported through it by others.

MOTHERHOOD

If yoga is a path towards knowing ourselves, motherhood is one of the most rigorous and rewarding of yoga practices. Our children are our most exacting teachers, knowing instinctively which buttons to push, while at the same time offering and asking for unconditional love. The way I am with my children is like a mirror that shows me the efficacy of my own yoga practice. Because my children seem to incite such a large range of responses from me, from deep love to anger, rapture to irritation, the quality of my presence is mirrored back clearly. Am I able to feel this moment fully, but then let it go? Or do I find myself contracting around my anger or irritation in an effort either to deny it or hold on to it? When we 'contract' in this way around physical or emotional pain, we allow the experience to become bigger than us, to define who we are. The same is true on the mat in a difficult pose. If in place of pushing through discomfort as if it weren't there, or focusing in on it and feeling overwhelmed, we expand our awareness to include all the other parts of ourselves – our lifted chest, our deep breathing, long spine, relaxed face – we remain bigger than the challenge. We feel it fully, then let it go. Practising yoga with an attitude of sensitive listening to create space in the body can help us create space in ourselves in our interactions off the mat too.

My children are a constant reminder that my physical yoga practice is not an end in itself, but a tool to live a vibrantly awake and engaged life.

SUPPORTING THE MENOPAUSE

Though menopause is technically 12 months after your final period, many women experience turbulent symptoms in the years up to it and beyond. The average age of menopause in the UK is 51, but symptoms can start up to ten years before (known as perimenopause), and continue for up to five years afterwards. Women may experience an erratic cycling of the hormones oestrogen, progesterone and testosterone that can lead to hot flushes, insomnia, fatigue, depression, irritability and anxiety. The menopause often goes hand-in-hand with pressures in our family lives, such as illness, ageing parents,

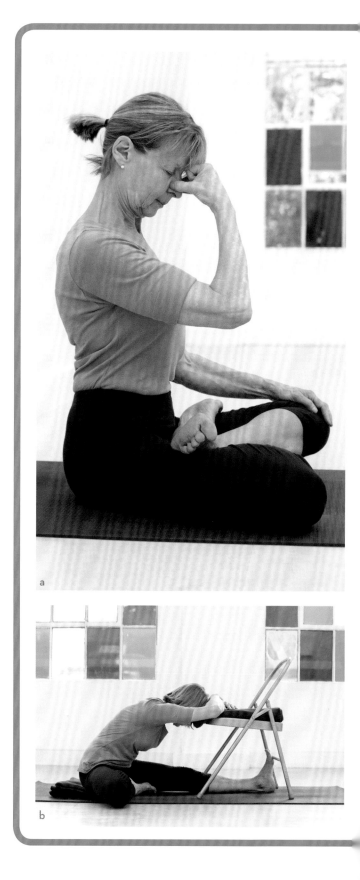

a

b

hot flushes

Nearly 70 per cent of British women experience hot flushes around menopause.[4] If these happen while we are asleep, night sweats can be so powerful that they wake us. Falling levels of oestrogen and other reproductive hormones are partly to blame, but stress, fatigue and intense periods of activity can also intensify these episodes. A yoga practice that is cooling and restorative, emphasising deep breathing, can help.

HELP FOR HOT FLUSHES:

1. Good breathing. Probably your most important and accessible tool is to remember to breathe well! Research has shown that breathing with deep, slow inhalations that fill up the belly followed by long, smooth, slow exhalations can stop hot flushes in their tracks and reduce frequency by 50 to 60 per cent.[5] More refined breathing techniques include alternate nostril breathing (*nadi shodhana* **(a)**, for instructions see page 168), which balances the hemispheres of the brain, soothing body and mind.

2. Supported forward bends. Practising these standing and seated, with your head resting on a bolster or chair **(b)**, helps cool the body and calm the nervous system.

3. Supported reclining poses. Reclining bound angle pose **(c)** (*supta baddha konasana*) and reclining hero pose (*supta virasana*; see page 121 picture **(a)**) allow the belly to soften and the chest to open so that your breathing is more effective.

4. Inversions. These support the neuroendocrine system by allowing fresh, oxygenated blood to flow to your head and neck and can help to either jump-start a sluggish system or calm an overexcited one. If you already regularly practise headstand and shoulder stand, you should continue unless you feel any strain. Some women find doing headstand against the wall (or hanging from wall ropes in class) with the soles of the feet together or legs wide apart is more soothing, likewise shoulder stand supported by bolsters and a chair (see page 122). If these poses aren't in your regular practice, a gentler inversion such as supported bridge pose **(d)** (*setu bandha sarvangasana*) over bolsters is a powerful alternative.

Research has shown that deep breathing can stop hot flushes.

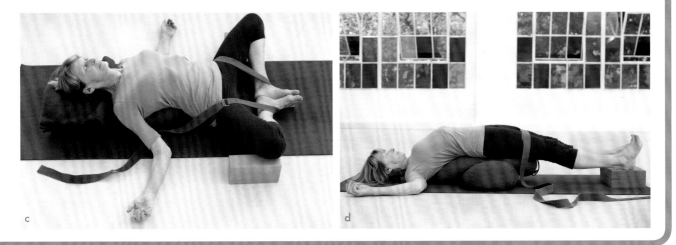

c

d

challenging teens or an empty nest. Our degree of stress has a profound effect on our bodies and may influence which menopausal symptoms we have, how severe they are and how long they go on for.

Yoga can be a lifeline for women at this stage, reducing stress, stabilising body temperature, boosting mood and helping support a positive self-image during the transition. It is also increasingly recognised that a spiritual component in our lives contributes to greater happiness and health. Ultimately, our yoga practice takes us to the very core of existence, and the radical perspective that we are all expansive, loving and spacious at this core. When we align ourselves with this potential, we are more open to welcoming both change and the unknown into our lives.

Fatigue

Tiredness is another common complaint around the menopause. Even women who have no other symptoms often feel that they lack vitality. This may be caused by depleted adrenals: the result of a stressful lifestyle coupled with the hormonal changes of menopause.

Try this: Begin your practice with supported reclining poses and forward bends, to help to pacify the adrenals and quieten the sympathetic ('fight or flight') nervous system. Then a well-rounded yoga practice including standing poses, backbends and twists will massage and stimulate the adrenal glands and replenish your energy levels.

Anxiety, depression and mood swings

Fluctuations in progesterone and oestrogen contribute to erratic moods, as also happens during puberty. Too much oestrogen can tip us into anxiety; too much progesterone leaves us susceptible to depression.

Try this: Backbends, especially if they are supported by props, such as inverted staff pose (*viparita dandasana*) over a chair (see right) bring a lightness to the body and improve breathing and circulation, all of which counter feelings of depression. Inversions: legs-up-the-wall pose (*viparita karani*) are soothing for the nervous system, helping to ground you when you feel as though you are losing control of your

environment. As before, if stronger inversions such as headstand and shoulder stand are part of your practice, continue with these also.

Reconnect and celebrate

How you feel about entering menopause in general, and getting older in particular, will also impact on your mood. Oestrogen is the hormone that makes us 'feminine', with thick hair, moist skin and a soft voice, so it is helpful to acknowledge a letting-go of that part of yourself in order to welcome the next phase of your life. Yoga reconnects you to what is going on inside at this moment, to help you feel who you are, rather than what society thinks you ought to be. Instead of mourning lost youth, this can be an invitation to tap into the richness, strength and freedom of this stage of your life.

AGEING

Yoga can help counteract the physical manifestations of ageing – keeping your joints and muscles moving freely, your organs supported and well-nourished with blood supply, and generally keeping you limber and self-reliant for longer. A yoga practice can be helpful for the common complaints of both arthritis and osteoporosis. For arthritis, do poses that encourage movement in your joints, very gently and without holding, to improve blood circulation, gain mobility and strengthen the surrounding ligaments and tissues. For osteoporosis, weight-bearing postures help to improve bone density, thereby preventing its onset, or reducing its effects if it is already present. Poses that are particularly beneficial include dog pose, most standing poses and in some

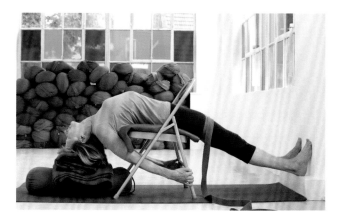

cases even handstand (see right) or upward-facing bow pose (*urdhva dhanurasana*) if you are up to it (and, if not, you can use props).

The physical side, of course, is only half the picture. Traditional Chinese medicine takes the view that a healthy woman experiences a 'second spring' after menopause. If she is well nourished and exercises appropriately, she can experience great vitality, clarity, energy, leadership and vision as she heads towards her sixties and beyond.

Nowadays, however, we revere youth above the wisdom and experience of age. When we are young, we have more energy and greater capacity to deal with stress – but for a reason. We are strong, but ignorant: we need that energy to make enough mistakes in order to learn and grow! As we get older – so long as we have been willing to learn from life – our wisdom allows us to direct our smaller reserves of energy sensitively and efficiently.

We may begin our yoga journey learning how to place ourselves in alignment in a pose, but the sensitivity that starts here in our body will grow over time and expand to include our heart and mind. This sensitivity is infinitely richer than the undirected buoyancy of youth. Once we finally elevate the wisdom of age above the energy of youth as a culture, it will also free us from our fear of change: plastic surgery to look younger, 'nip and tuck' post-elective C-section to look as if we have never had a baby will no longer be desirable. Instead we can embrace change – including growing older – as the greatest vehicle we have for genuine transformation and growth.

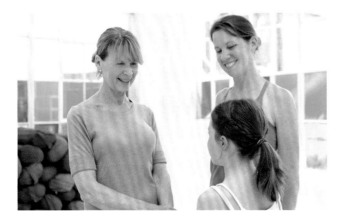

weight bearing postures help to improve bone density, preventing the onset or reducing the effect of osteoporosis

yoga *for relationships*

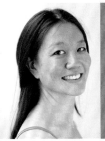

'The purpose of yoga is to facilitate the profound inner relaxation that accompanies fearlessness. The release from fear is what finally precipitates the full flowering of love. In this state you will love what you see in others, and others will love you for having been seen' — Erich Schiffmann[1]

BY MIMI KUO-DEEMER

Erich Schiffmann was my first yoga teacher. He told me that yoga would change the way I live and see life. I had no idea what he meant, but I was ready for something to shift my unhealthy, asthmatic state that often left me in an unhappy and anxious frame of mind. It was only years later that I realised what he was saying – that yoga had an effect far beyond its physical benefits.

Many of us come to yoga because we have heard it can help us physically and give us a chance to relax. It was only by doing yoga that I discovered that it also unveiled how the mind works. The process of breathing deeply, moving mindfully and sitting quietly in meditation gave me a perspective on all the irrelevant narratives that went on in my head; it also offered me a way of stepping out of them. In time, I found that when I grew quieter in my own mental space, this had a positive effect on my relationships with others.

Indeed, the physical practice is just one of many doorways into a profound spiritual tradition. We may be able to do 108 sun salutations or put our leg behind our head, but, in the words of the yoga teacher and writer Donna Farhi, 'our spiritual fitness can be tested only in relationship to others.'[2]

Many of the problems we have in relationships stem from acting without thinking. Whether it be down to our personal frustrations on that particular day or misunderstandings or hurts we have experienced from the past – our accumulated conditioning can lead us to think unpleasant things about people or to say and do things that we regret. In yoga, our repeated patterns of

behaviour – whether positive or negative, and whether consciously intended or not – are known as *samskaras* (see page 105).

A yoga practice offers us time to pause for breath and live in our bodies in a more mindful way. When we are present in a non-judgemental way, we can begin to see more clearly, rather than through the lens of past experiences or anxieties about the future. This can allow many of our *samskaras* (conditioned habits) to surface. We can then begin to work to keep those that serve us well – such as listening before jumping to conclusions – and discard or shift the ones that we're better off without, such as knee-jerk reactions. This gradual yet radical process of self-acceptance can be quite scary when we first try it out. Indeed, when we see what's happening inside our minds it's not always pretty! The effort, however, is worth it.

When we begin to act from a more contemplative mindset, the greatest beneficiaries are our friends, family, colleagues and even strangers. We are much less likely to judge or blame them and they may, in turn, be less likely to judge us.

To make the challenge of managing our relationships a little easier, the ancient yogic texts offer us four principles for living – the *brahmavihara*. They are approaches to how we can interact with others in a way that causes us the least mental turmoil. Because they often go against our conditioning, they may not be the easiest of paths; but that's the great strength of yoga practice – little by little it begins to change us.

'Our spiritual fitness
can be tested only
in relationship
to others.'

the four-part plan for better relationships

The *brahmavihara* make up my favourite of all the *Yoga Sutras*, written by the sage Patanjali 2,000 years ago. *Sutra* (1.33) reads...

'Maitri karuna mudita upekshanam sukha duhka punya apunya vishayanam bhavanatah chitta prasadanam'

...which translates as 'Consciousness [i.e. the busy mind] settles when we radiate friendliness, compassion, delight and equanimity toward all things, whether pleasant, painful, good or bad.'[3]

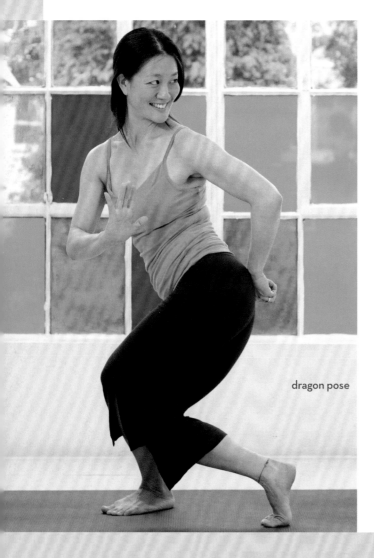

dragon pose

THE BRAHMAVIHARA OR 'FOUR ATTITUDES':

1. *Maitri* – friendliness towards the joyful

This first *brahmavihara* seems fairly straightforward – happiness is a quality we all strive for. In reality, however, other people's happiness is often a challenge to accept. To celebrate someone else's joy rather than be envious or disapproving often requires us to set aside our own opinions and expectations and simply see it as a source of inspiration.

2. *Karuna* – compassion for those who are suffering

When we are unhappy, the slightest recognition of our suffering by someone else – a subtle smile, a quick email – fills us with gratitude. Someone is seeing us as we are and not judging us. To extend compassion to someone who is having a hard time moves us out of a space of indifference or frustration and into a place of love.

Again, this idea may sound simple, but who hasn't become annoyed with their perpetually grumpy colleague, or felt superior to a friend going through a break-up because we've worked through hard times in a relationship and come out stronger?

Rather than letting someone else's unhappiness became a source of frustration, let it become a source of recognition or caring. This can be as simple as extending a helpful thought to someone in need, or awakening the practice of compassion into the charitable giving of money, resources and time.

There's a fine line between compassion and commiseration, however. It's important to be empathetic, but when one person starts telling a difficult and sad story, sometimes we feel compelled to start telling our own tragic saga. Sometimes we hear of a dilemma and feel obliged to offer strategies to fix it. Compassion is about offering a helping hand and lending a friendly ear.

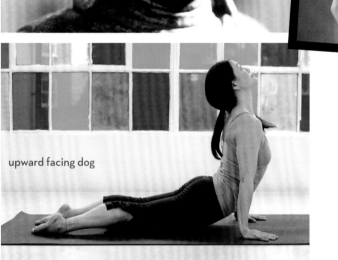

upward facing dog

3. *Mudita* – delight in the good fortune and good qualities of others

When someone has been rewarded – with a pay rise or an accolade – we can sometimes be quick to question whether they deserve it. Or when we meet a person who seems really nice and well-intentioned, we can sometimes doubt their sincerity. But we don't have to react that way. We can celebrate another person's good achievements and virtues. If we are able to feel genuine delight for someone else's good qualities, it generates less envy and more positivity.

4. *Upekshanam* – equanimity towards others' faults and shortcomings

If someone messes up, it's easy to look down on them. But imagine it's you on the receiving end. Isn't it nicer to have your good qualities recognised than have your bad habits picked apart?

In the *brahmavihara*, Patanjali offers us ways of seeing and interacting with other people that will help us stay calm. Maintaining our peace of mind when someone has wronged us is perhaps the biggest task of all. If we are eaten up with anger or hatred towards another person, it only makes us more miserable. Since the bad deed is already done, being angry only wastes energy. A far better use of our mental and emotional resources is to reframe that experience for ourselves (so much easier said than done, but Patanjali urges us to try). The hardest task is when we are faced with violent atrocities. Of course we shouldn't stand back and watch a bad situation unfold if it's within our power to change it. But we can choose our perspective. On the one hand we can be filled with loathing and say, 'This person is evil and should face the direst consequences,' but on the other hand, yoga would say that what caused this person to commit these atrocities was an accumulation of negative or abusive experiences. Hating the deed rather than the person allows us to retain our humanity and build relationships rather than pile up enemies. I find it helpful to think that when Patanjali's *Yoga Sutras* were written, the ancient yogis were as flawed and challenged at calming themselves down as I may be; this makes friendliness, compassion, delight and equanimity in the face of all things good, bad, happy and unhappy sound like a reasonable endeavour.

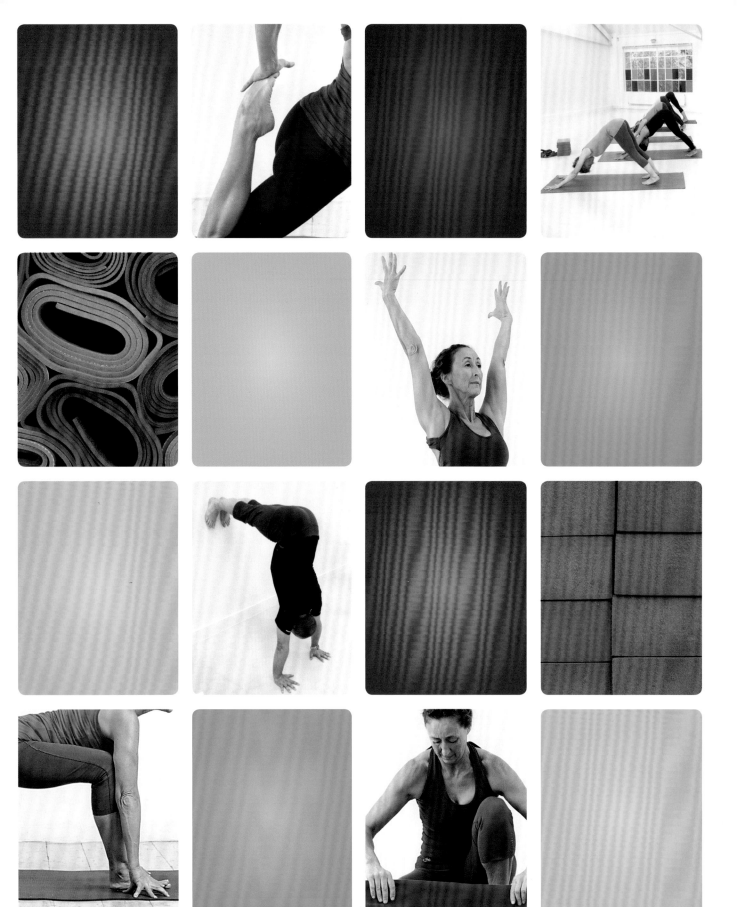

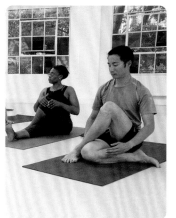

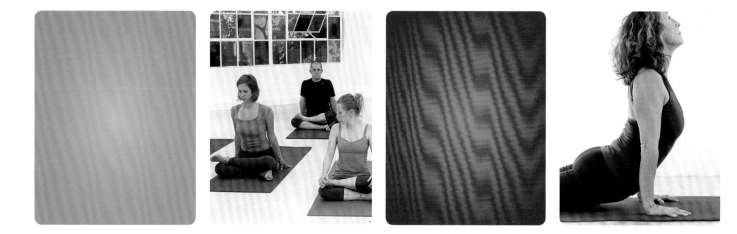

the practice

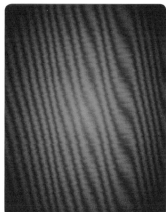

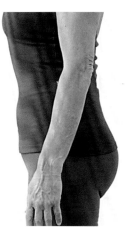

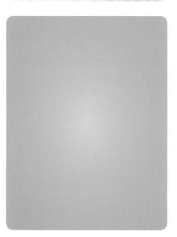

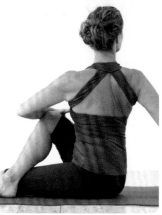

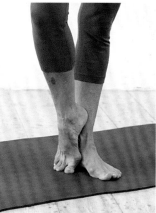

prepare to practise

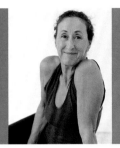

Before you begin the sequences on the following pages – or any yoga practice – applying some basic principles of alignment will help you practise safely and feel good

BY BRIDGET WOODS-KRAMER

The three 20-minute sequences on the following pages are designed to be practised individually as well as one after the other. The morning sequence is dynamic and energising, the midday strengthening and focusing and the evening calming and relaxing. Of course they can be done at other times of day, depending on the energetic effect you are looking for. If you are joining up two or more sequences, please do them in numerical order (i.e. follow 1 with 2 and/or 3 but not 1 after 2 or 3) so you begin with the most dynamic first. Remember also to omit final relaxation poses and practise only the relaxation at the end of your last sequence. Feel free to hold the poses longer than indicated, just make sure that whatever you do on the right side of the body, you repeat on the left.

Not all poses have specific English and Sanskrit names. We have named the most common ones where they first appear. As for how to breathe, we use *ujjayi* breath (see page 168) apart from during meditation and relaxation, or where another breath exercise is given. When practising at home omit inversions (i.e. going upside down) if you have very high or low blood pressure, or have neck injuries or glaucoma or if you are on your menstrual cycle. In the following sequences, there are two inversions – half handstand (midday – pose 4d) and legs-up-the-wall (evening – pose 4a). Instead, take downward facing dog and legs-up-the-wall without a bolster or cushion respectively. If you feel pain or dizziness at any point, come into child's pose or lie on your back. Please consult your doctor before starting yoga practice. In a class setting always advise your teacher if you have any health concerns.

TEN THINGS TO KNOW BEFORE YOU START

Here are some basic principles of alignment to observe in yoga so that we can practise safely and our energy can flow in an optimum way.

1. Root down through four corners of feet

This is key for any standing pose. The easiest way to experience this is by standing with feet hip-width apart and parallel. Spread the toes and press all four corners of each foot into the floor. Remember this connection in all standing poses – especially triangle and warrior 2, where it's easy for the weight to collapse into the inner edge of the foot.

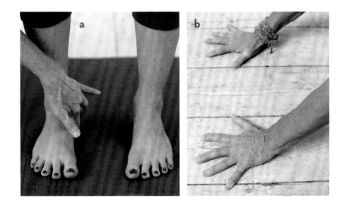

Watch point: By 'feet parallel' we don't mean lining the outer or inner edges up. Instead, imagine on each foot a line running between the second and third toes to the centre of the ankle. Place these lines parallel. This makes for correct alignment whatever shape your feet are. Keep the outer heel rooted so you can lift through the inner arches of the foot. **(a)**

2. Spread the hands broadly

In poses where the weight is in your hands (such as downward facing dog, plank, handstand) spread the fingers wide. Line the creases of the wrists up with the front edge of the mat. Look for an even crease along the wrist **(b)**. Press down through the knuckles, the base of the index finger, base of the thumb, little finger and outer palm. Keeping the knuckles grounded, root through the ends of your finger pads. As you root the hands, draw up from there into the shoulders, creating a sense of stability and feeling the integration of the arms into the shoulder joint. In downward facing dog, you should feel the centre of your palm lifting and the underside of your forearm drawing away from the floor.
Watch point: Make sure that the base of the index finger stays grounded – it will want to lift!

3. Root before you rise

Rooting – the feeling of pushing roots down into the earth from your foundation – gives stability to any reaching, rising, bending or twisting action that follows. In standing poses, the foundation is our legs. Think of the rooting action beginning deep in the core of the lower belly (between the pubic bone and navel **(d)**) and travelling down through strong legs and steady feet. In sitting poses, manually turn the flesh of each thigh in to feel the sitbones broaden at the back **(c)**, giving you a wider foundation and maintaining the natural curve in the lower back. Then root down through your sitbones into the floor.

4. Stack the joints

Aligning the joints vertically on top of each other (see mountain pose, page 140) ensures that our weight travels in a straight line down into the floor, protecting the joints. No joint is sticking out or collapsing in awkwardly or taking more than its fair share of weight.
— **Stack tops of shoulders over elbows, and elbows over wrists** e.g. handstand, all fours, plank, side plank, low lunge **(e)**.
— **Stack pelvis, knees and ankles** e.g. mountain pose, tree pose (page 141).
— **Stack bent knee over ankle** e.g. warrior 1, warrior 2, chair pose, extended side angle. Make sure the knee doesn't collapse in or out. It should line up with the centre of the foot **(e)**.
Watch point: When we extend out through the arms and legs, it's easy to overextend through the joints rather than stretching out through the muscles. First draw the limbs in to their sockets to stabilise the joints.

5. Keep length in the spine

There are two natural curves (i.e. where the vertebra move into the body), one in the lower back (the lumbar spine) and the other in the neck (cervical spine). When we hunch forwards – at our desks, slouching back into soft sofas or even in yoga, trying too hard to reach our toes – not only do we lose the spine's natural curves but

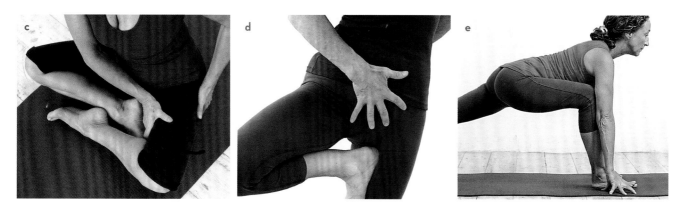

we also put pressure on the discs, causing them to protrude. These curves are crucial for keeping the back strong and healthy. Yoga should bring them back into balance so our spine stays strong. If we have a tendency to hunch, as well as putting pressure on the discs, it tightens the upper back, pulls our shoulders forward, tightens the chest muscles and so restricts the breath – our life force – draining our energy. All good arguments for keeping the spine flexible and healthy.

Watch point: When bending forward, do so from the hip crease, not lower back **(f)**. Most lower back injuries occur from bending down incorrectly.

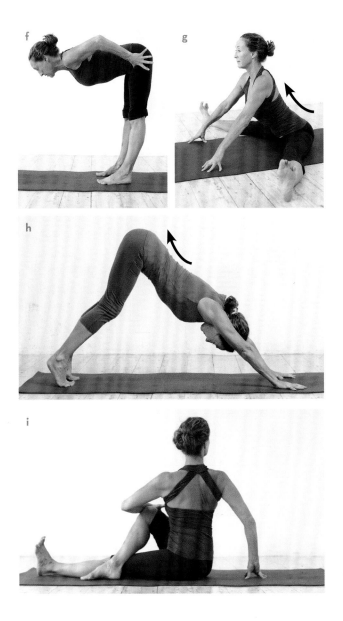

— **Spine long in seated forward bends:** First find the curve in the lower back. For this to happen, the top of your sacrum (the flat bone at the base of the spine) needs to lift up and in towards the spine, bringing a curve to the lower back **(g)**. Then the thighs will ground. One action to enhance this is manually turning the upper thighs in (see **(c)**). If your legs and back are tight, you may need to sit higher on a block or cushion.

Watch point: Remember 'curve before extension' in all seated forward bends and to bend from the hip crease not the lower back.

— **Spine long in standing forward bends:** If your hamstrings are tight, bend the knees first. Tilt your sitbones higher in the air to feel the slight curve in the lower back. If you can't reach the floor without rounding, place blocks under the hands.

Watch point: In downward facing dog keep the curve in the lumbar spine by tilting the pelvis and lifting the sitbones to extend back **(h)**. Only then try straightening the legs.

6. Keep the core engaged

The lower belly should be engaged – but not rock hard – throughout the practice, except in relaxation. To feel this engagement, follow the instructions for the pelvis in mountain pose (page 140). This will also lift the pelvic floor, engaging *mula bandha* (page 170).

7. Twist from your core

It's tempting in any twist to lead with the head, but don't. Nor should a twist start from the waist. It originates from the lower belly (the area level with the second chakra between pubic bone and navel). Your head should be the last part of you to turn **(i)**.

Before you start to twist, root down through your foundation – whether it's your sitbones in a seated twist or your legs in a standing twist – and then take your attention to the back of the body, to the side you are turning away from. Breathe into that lung, feel it inflating in the back and begin to move that side of the body around. This will give you the feeling of the inner body twisting too. All the time keep length and space in the torso and shoulder blades drawing back.

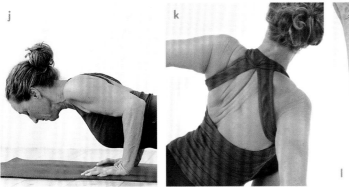

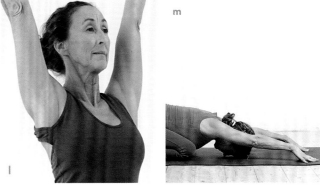

8. Shoulders back and heart lifted

In all poses, remember to keep the sides of the torso long and the heart lifted as you shrug the shoulder blades down the back (j, k, l, m, o). Don't let the lower ribs stick out as you do this. Consciously breathing into the back ribs will help counteract this tendency.

Watch point: Even in child's pose remember to keep the shoulder blades on the back (m).

9. Lengthen the sides of the neck

The neck is an extension of your spine, so remember to lengthen here too in all poses. Think of the length as being through the sides of the neck rather than the front or back – dropping the head forward flattens the natural curve, while sticking the chin out compresses the cervical vertebrae. Take the upper palate and ears back so that the head sits on top of the neck – and remember that the neck also has a gentle curve. The chin is lifted slightly, but not jutting forward. If turning the neck sideways to look up (as in triangle pose) feels painful in any way, look straight ahead instead.

Watch point: In poses such as upward facing dog and cobra, it's easy stick out the chin too much, as it makes us feel like we are lifting higher (n). In fact the lift begins in the bottom of the heart. Lift the heart and then lift the gaze from the eyes (o).

10. Look after your knees

The knee is a relatively weak and unstable joint, but one that nevertheless has a lot of work to do. It's no

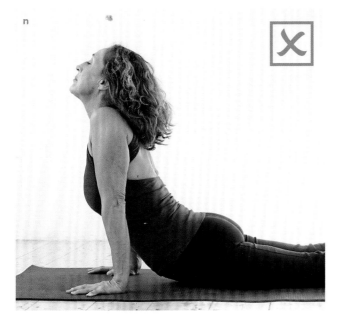

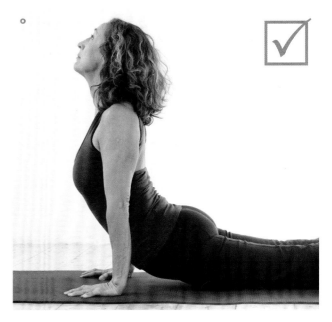

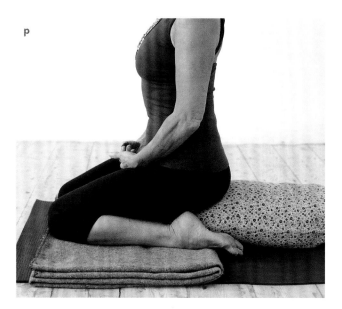

p

surprise that knee injuries are common. If you know you have tight hips (for example, if your knees are high off the ground when you sit cross-legged), it's easy to misalign the knees. So take care in hip openers such as firelog and pigeon (page 158–9). Never work through pain in your knee. Ease off and focus on the alignment in your hips.

— **Kneeling:** If kneeling feels too hard on the kneecap, place a folded towel or blanket underneath, or create a fold in the mat for double thickness. Some poses such as hero pose **(p)** and child's pose involve sitting with bent knees on or between the heels. If knee issues create difficulty for you here, place a folded blanket or blocks under your bottom, as shown.

props – and how to use them

Props are used to enhance alignment and to help you into a pose, but they shouldn't become a crutch.

Strap or belt: This adds length to arms – for example, to prevent hunching in a seated forward bend or to make sure we don't overextend the shoulder joint when tight hips and legs stop us being able to reach our toes.

It can also be used to provide stability and support: for example, in the restorative yoga pose supported bridge (page 79). Here, the thighs are bound together with a strap so that you can totally relax into the pose.

Bolsters: These are used mainly in restorative poses for greater support and relaxation.

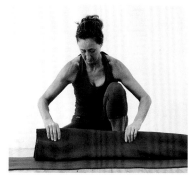

Blankets: A folded blanket, towel or yoga mat can add extra cushioning and height where you need it. In *savasana* (final relaxation) take a towel and concertina-fold from the long edge about five times (see above). Lie down with one end of the towel at your tailbone and the other folded into a pleat to support the neck as shown right. This gives a greater opening in the chest as you relax.

Blocks: Placed under the sitbones, these can help you sit higher, which is useful if sitting causes the back to round. They can also give you something to ground to – under the bent-leg thigh in pigeon, for example, or beneath the hands in a standing forward bend if you can't reach the floor.

Eye bags: These can deepen final relaxation by blocking out the light. The weight of the bag helps relax the nervous system.

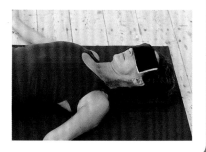

— **Standing:** If you are very flexible, check that you are not locking the knees back too far when the legs are straight, especially in poses such as wide legged forward bend **(q)**. If you feel pressure in the back of the knees, soften them a little, engage the calf muscles and lift the kneecaps.

When the knee is bent in standing poses (such as warrior 2, lunge and extended side angle) keep it directly above the ankle and lined up over the centre of the foot as before. The weight should not go forward into the knees. To avoid this, draw back into the hip.

— **Sitting:** Some poses involve the weight from another part of your body being placed on your bent knee (for instance, pigeon **(r)**, firelog). If you have had a knee injury or experience any pain in the knee, ask your teacher for modification. When doing the sequences in this book, follow the 'knee variation' alternatives. Pictures **(s)** and **(t)** are both good pigeon alternatives.

AWARENESS: YOUR CONSTANT COMPANION

Yoga builds strength and flexibility, but ultimately it's about becoming more aware. Awareness is key if we are to get the most out of a practice and avoid injury.

So as you practise remember to keep your attention on each breath as you ground through your foundation. This will anchor you in the present moment and connect you with what's going on in your body right now – whether a pose feels right, whether you can go deeper or whether you need to ease off. It's when we move unconsciously that we are most prone to injury.

When we become more aware of the body, we start to become more aware of what is good for it and what makes us feel better in our own skin. Over time, and with practice, that awareness broadens so that we become more aware of the choices that make us feel better mentally and emotionally. In this way a regular yoga practice impacts positively on our lives off the mat too.

Awareness is also the key component of a meditation practice. So by practising yoga with awareness, you are engaging in a moving meditation.

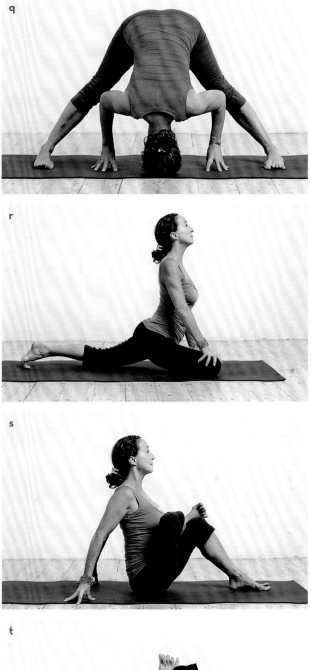

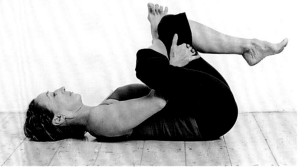

mountain pose – (tadasana)
the one pose you really need to know

It is said that this simple standing pose contains all the important alignment points for every other yoga pose, so it's worth taking a little time to learn to set it up.

1. FEET

The first thing to set up correctly in any pose is the foundation – the part of you that is in contact with the floor.

Stand at the front of the mat, with feet parallel and hip-width apart. Classical alignment teaches standing with feet together. However, taking them a little wider allows for greater ease of movement.

Press all four corners of the feet into the floor, starting with the base of the big toe, followed by the inner heel, base of the little toe and the outer heel. This makes a difference to how the leg engages. The inner arch of the foot lifts and the calf draws back and up.

2. KNEES

Once you have set up the feet, soften the knees and line them up directly over the ankles. Then draw the kneecaps up, engaging the thighs.

3. PELVIS

Stack the tops of the thigh bones over the knees. For most of us this means drawing the tops of the thighs back slightly. Do this by rotating the upper thighs inwards, moving them back and widening them apart, deepening the curve in the lower back (so that your bottom sticks out).

Now balance this action by scooping the tailbone (coccyx) down (your bottom comes back in a little) but without letting the thighs push forwards again. A gentle natural curve should remain in the lower back. In doing this you should also feel a lift in the pelvic floor (*mula bandha*, see page 170) and the muscles of the lower belly engage.

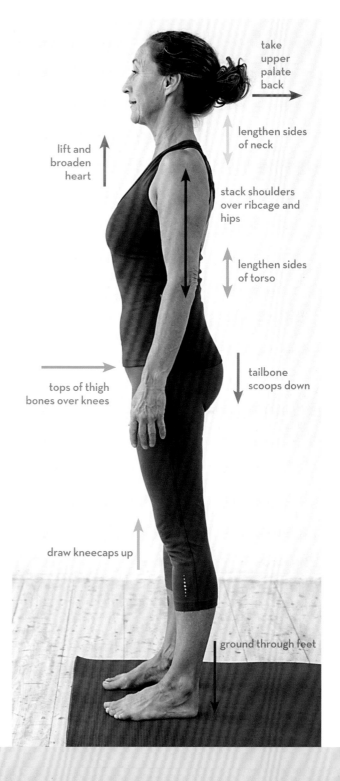

take upper palate back

lengthen sides of neck

lift and broaden heart

stack shoulders over ribcage and hips

lengthen sides of torso

tailbone scoops down

tops of thigh bones over knees

draw kneecaps up

ground through feet

Watch point: If you look side-on in a mirror you should be able to see that the centre of the thigh lines up with the centre of the knee and the ankle.

4. TORSO

Now that you have grounded through your legs, lengthen up through your spine and the sides of your torso, leaving space in the armpits. Keep the heart lifted and open: think of the heart space broadening in all directions – front, back and out to the sides.

Throughout the practice, feel length and space – a brightness – in the inner body. This is an area that is so often compressed by modern desk- based life.

5. SHOULDERS

Now stack the shoulders and ribcage over the pelvis. Keeping the sides of the torso long and armpits lifted, take the head of the arm bones (i.e. the tops of the shoulders) back. Feel the bottom tips of the shoulder blades drawing towards each other and flowing down the back. Breathe into the back ribs.

6. HEAD AND NECK

Lengthen the sides of the neck. Take the upper palate and ears back to so that the head sits on top of the cervical spine. The chin is slightly lifted, but not sticking out, and there is a gentle curve in the back of the neck.

TRY THIS: FIND THE ALIGNMENT OF MOUNTAIN POSE IN...

— **Plank (page 147):** Rooting back through the legs, turn the tops of the thighs in and back. With the sacrum broad, lengthen the tailbone to the heels, engaging the lower belly and pelvic floor. Draw the shoulder blades back, keep the collarbones broad and your gaze slightly forwards.

— *Chaturanga dandasana* **(push-up, page 148):** As above, but be especially mindful of keeping the head of the arm bones back and the heart and collarbones broad as you lower. It's a common misconception that *chaturanga* is all about arm strength. Strongly rooting back through the legs and engaging the core – just as you did while standing in mountain pose – distributes the weight more evenly throughout the body, not just through the arms.

— **Single leg balances, e.g. tree pose (below) and dancer (page 154):** Stacking the joints, ankles, knees and pelvis, start to shift your weight to the supporting leg, root down from the core of the pelvis into the foundation, and allow the spine to lengthen upwards. Fix your gaze on a non-moving point and find a steadiness of breath. In tree pose, press your bent-leg foot and thigh together with equal pressure to bring an inner stability (see below). In dancer, your foot and hand press together creating stability. Over time you should be able to keep your gaze steady and widen your awareness to the outer corner of your eyes and the sides of the room. You are centred yet spacious.

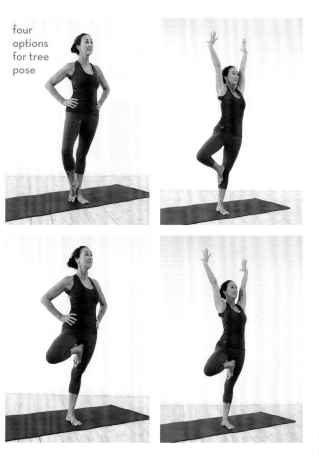

four options for tree pose

morning sequence – energising + awakening

BY BRIDGET WOODS-KRAMER

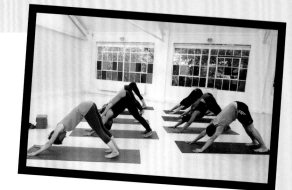

you can also follow this
sequence on the DVD

FOCUS: Awakening the spine, moving the breath and body, building strength in arms, legs and core.

FLOW: We start lying down with leg stretches, then move to all fours, gently warming up the spine by rounding and arching the back. Dynamic sun salutations flow into push-ups, core work, leg-strengthening warrior and triangle poses to help you meet the day with strength and brightness.

YOU WILL NEED: A yoga strap (a belt or long scarf will also do the job). A cushion under your buttocks if you find it hard to sit tall with a straight spine.

For a shorter ten-minute practice do:
2) Awakening
6) Building Heat
12) Strong Legs, Open Heart (starting from **d**)

1. MOVING THE BREATH

seated ujjayi breathing

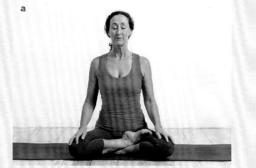

a. Sit cross-legged, hands on knees. Keep gaze soft. *Ujjayi* breathing (see page 168) for about a minute.

2. AWAKENING

reclining leg stretches

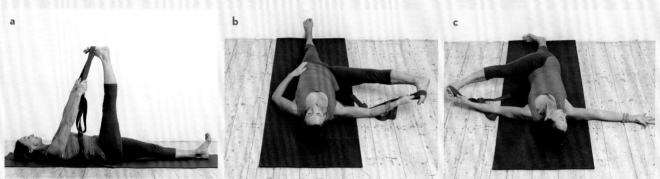

a. Lie with feet flat (against wall if possible). Take belt in both hands and around ball of right foot. Raise right leg to sky.

Hold for five breaths [reclining hand-to-big-toe pose, *supta padangusthasana*]

b. Take belt in right hand. Release right leg out to right. Left foot flexed, left thigh grounded, both shoulders on the ground. Hold for five breaths.

c. Take belt in left hand. Extend right leg across body. Hold for five breaths. *Repeat sequence using other leg.*

3. AWAKENING THE SPINE

cat/cow

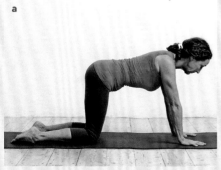

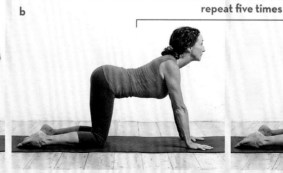

repeat five times

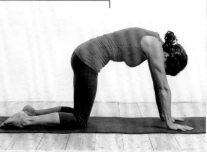

a. Come on to all fours, toes pointed. Hands spread below shoulders. Knees below hips.

b. Inhale, tilt tailbone to sky. Shoulders back, arch back. Look forwards. [cow]

c. Exhale, scoop tailbone under. Round the back, tuck the chin in. [cat] *Repeat b and c five times.*

4. RISING

downward facing dog to standing

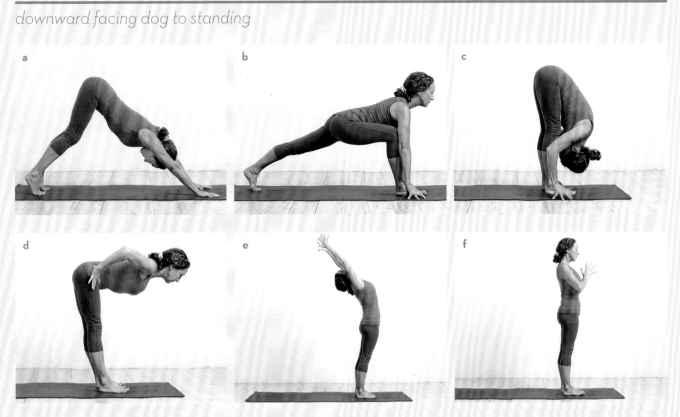

a

b

c

d

e

f

a. From all fours, take knees back 5cm (2in). Tuck toes under, lift hips, stretch back. Lengthen spine, knees bent. Let the head dangle; stay for five breaths. [downward facing dog, *adho mukha svanasana*]

b. Inhale, step right foot forwards to lunge. Look forwards. Stretch through back heel.

c. Exhale, left foot forwards. Feet hip-width apart. Bow down, chin to shin. [standing forward bend, *uttanasana*]

d. Inhale, hands to hips. Exhale, root down through legs.

e. Lengthen spine. Inhale, come up with flat back. Raise arms overhead.

f. Exhale, draw hands in prayer. Remember your *ujjayi* breath.

5. WARMING UP

sun salutation with baby cobra (j)

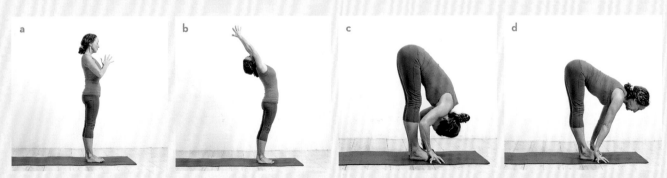

a

b

c

d

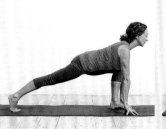
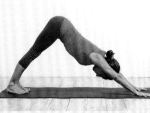
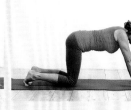
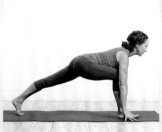

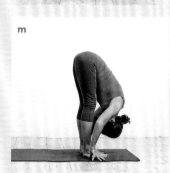
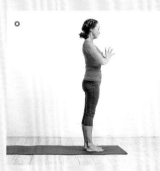
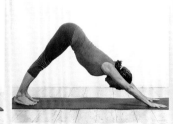

a. Begin in mountain pose with hands in prayer if you want. Feet hip-width apart, legs strong, hands by sides, shoulders back. [mountain pose, *tadasana*]

b. Inhale, arms to sky, look up.

c. Exhale, hinge at the hips, bend forward and down. Fingertips next to toes.

d. Inhale, look up. Chest open, heart forward, lengthen spine. [standing half forward bend, *ardha uttanasana*]

e. Exhale, step right leg back to low lunge, look ahead. Inhale, lengthen side body.

f. Exhale, take left leg back to downward facing dog. Keeping arms straight, root down from heart to floor. Moving tops of thighs back, straighten legs

g. Inhale on to all fours.

h. Exhale, bend elbows back. Lower chest between hands.

i. Continuing your exhale, lower body to floor. Chest between hands.

j. Inhale, point toes, draw hands back, shoulders back. Lift chest, keeping lower ribs on floor. [baby cobra, *bhujangasana*]

k. Exhale, root down through hands. Lift hips to downward facing dog.

l. Inhale, step right leg forward, look ahead. Extend through back leg.

m. Exhale, step left leg forward. Feet hip-width apart. Bow down, legs straight if possible.

n. Root down through legs. Inhale, come up, spine long. Raise arms overhead, look up.

o. Exhale, hands in prayer at heart. [equal standing pose, *samastithi*]

Repeat sequence, this time stepping left leg back at **e** *and left leg forwards at* **l** *so you work both sides of body.*

sun salutation with three-legged dog (l) to twisting lunge (n)

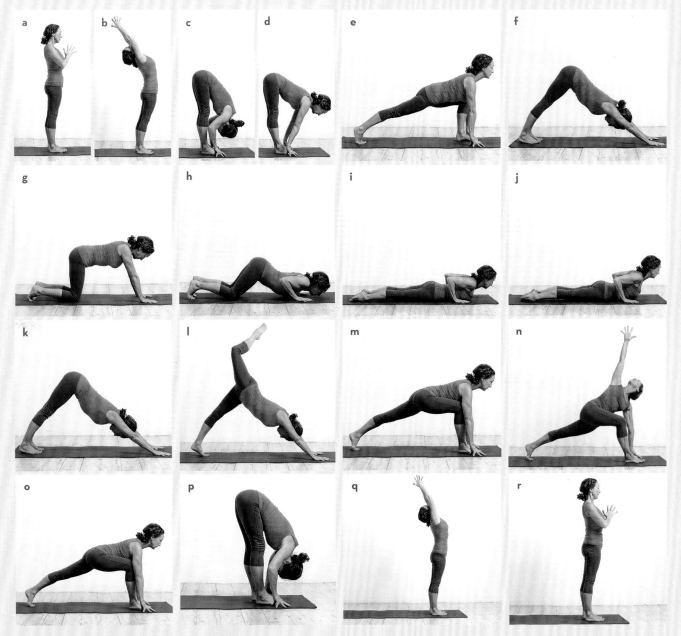

This sequence starts exactly like the previous one up to k (downward facing dog), and then adds three legged dog and a twisting lunge. We have shown you the poses in full above. For text instructions up to k please see sequence 5.

l. Inhale, right leg to sky. Bend knee, open right hip to sky. Hold for three breaths.

m. Exhale, right foot forwards.

n. Inhale, lengthen spine. Exhale, turn belly, ribs and chest to the right, raise right arm and look up. Hold for five breaths.

o. Exhale, hand back down.

p. Inhale, step the back leg forward. Exhale, bow down, straighten legs.

q. Root down through the legs. Inhale, come up with flat back. Raise arms, look up.

r. Exhale, hands in prayer in front of heart.

Repeat entire sequence on other side of body, leading with left leg this time.

7. TONING LEGS AND ARMS

a) mountain pose, b) chair pose, f) high lunge, g) plank, h–j) kneeling push-ups, l) cobra

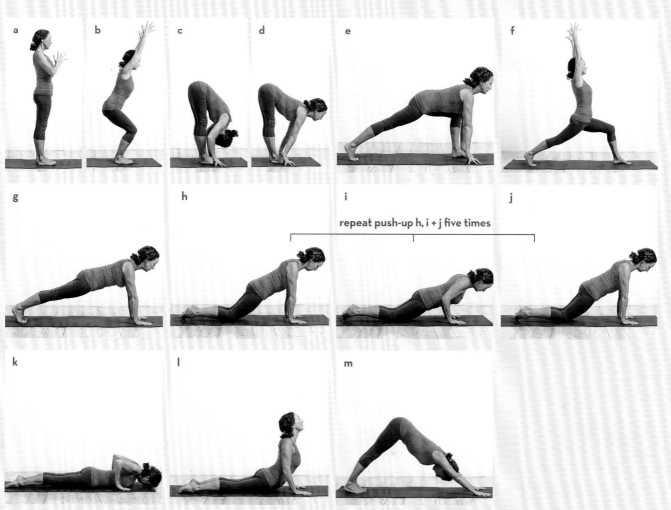

repeat push-up h, i + j five times

a. Begin in mountain pose with hands in prayer if desired.

b. Sink buttocks down. Keep knees above ankles. Inhale, stretch arms up. Hold for five breaths. [chair pose, *utkatasana*]

c. Exhale, bow down. Fingertips in line with toes. Straighten legs if possible.

d. Inhale as you look up. Straighten spine, shoulders back.

e. Exhale, right leg back to lunge. Keep back leg steady.

f. Inhale, bring torso vertical. Back leg steady, arms up. Hold for five breaths. [high lunge]

g. Exhale, hands to floor. Shoulders stay over wrists. Step left leg back. [plank pose]

h. Inhale, drop knees to floor. Toes tucked, shoulders back. Scoop tailbone under.

i. Keeping straight line from knees to shoulders, exhale and bend elbows. Lower chest halfway down, keep back of neck long. [kneeling push-up]

j. Push up strongly onto all fours. *Repeat push-up h–j five times.*

k. Lower body to floor. Lengthen back though legs, point toes.

l. Draw back through hands. Inhale, peel chest and ribs higher this time for full cobra. Elbows in, shoulders back.

m. Grounding through hands, exhale, lift hips for downward facing dog. Spine long, knees bent if needed.

Repeat sequence from f, taking high lunge on the other side by stepping the right foot forwards from downward facing dog.

8. WORKING ARMS AND CORE

nose-to-knee planks

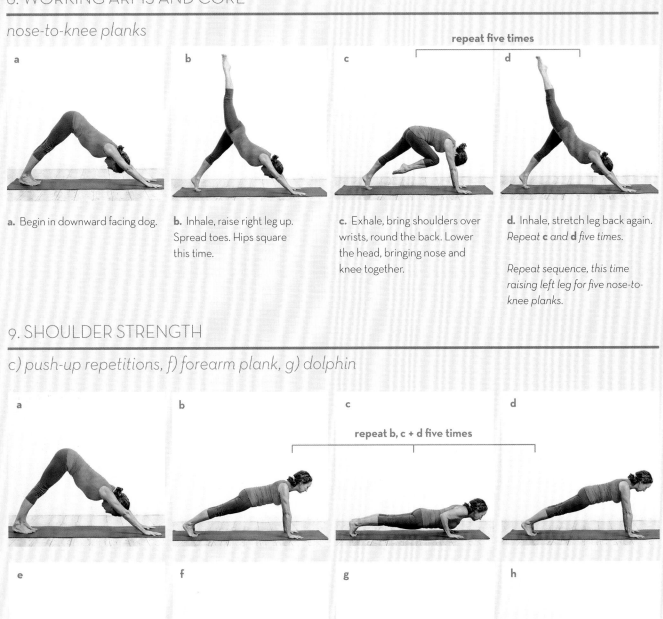

repeat five times

a. Begin in downward facing dog.

b. Inhale, raise right leg up. Spread toes. Hips square this time.

c. Exhale, bring shoulders over wrists, round the back. Lower the head, bringing nose and knee together.

d. Inhale, stretch leg back again. *Repeat **c** and **d** five times.*

Repeat sequence, this time raising left leg for five nose-to-knee planks.

9. SHOULDER STRENGTH

c) push-up repetitions, f) forearm plank, g) dolphin

repeat b, c + d five times

a. Begin in downward facing dog.

b. Inhale into plank, bringing shoulders over wrists. Extend back through heels.

c. Exhale, lower chest to elbow height. Keep front of shoulders lifted away from floor. Thighs and knees off floor. [push-up/four-limbed staff pose, *chaturanga dandasana*]

d. Inhale, push back up to plank. *Repeat **b**, **c** and **d** five times*

LESS CHALLENGING OPTION: Kneeling push-up as before (see 7h–j)

e. Exhale, lower body flat to floor. Toes tucked under this time.

f. Come onto forearms, elbows directly under shoulders. Lift knees and thighs. Scoop tailbone under, root back through legs. Hold for five breaths. [forearm plank]

g. Walk feet in towards hands. Hold for five breaths, keeping neck relaxed. [dolphin pose]

h. With knees slightly bent, exhale and press hands into floor. Inhale, lift forearms up. Straighten arms and legs to downward facing dog.

10. TONING THE SIDE WAIST

side plank

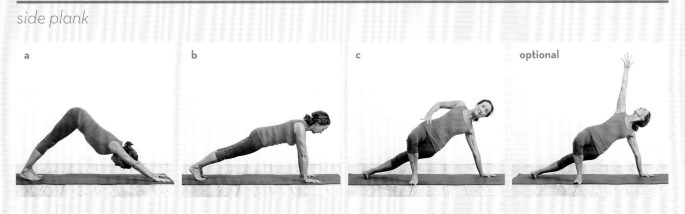

a

b

c

optional

a. Begin in downward facing dog.

b. Inhale into plank, shoulders over wrists.

c. Exhale, step right foot halfway to hands. Turn toes out to '3 o' clock' (when doing second side, left foot to '9 o' clock'). Place right hand on right hip. Come on to outside edge of left foot. Turn hips, shoulders to side of mat. Look up over shoulder for three to five breaths. [side plank, *vasisthasana*]

OPTIONAL CHALLENGE: Raise top arm, look at hand.

Repeat sequence on other side.

11. RESTING

child's pose

a. Sit back on the heels, point toes. Big toes together, knees wide. Forehead to floor, arms in front. Hold for five breaths. [child's pose, *balasana*]

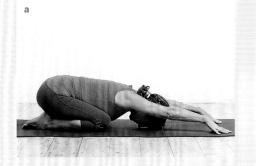

a

d) warrior 2, e) extended side angle, g) triangle, i) wide-legged forward bend, o) chair pose

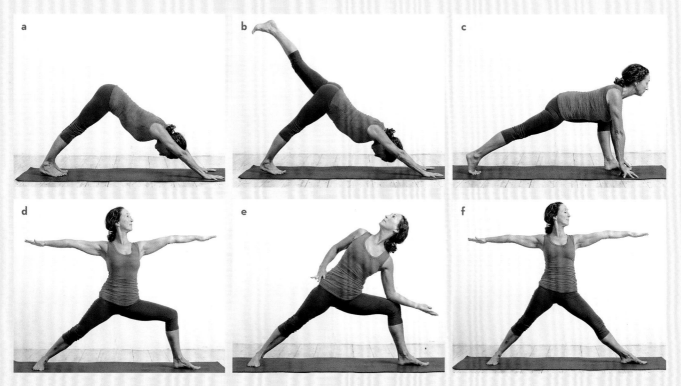

a. Begin in downward facing dog.

b. Leading with left leg first this time, inhale and raise left foot to sky.

c. Exhale, step left foot between hands, look ahead. Extend out through back heel.

d. Turn back foot flat and parallel to back of mat. Bend front knee to 90 degrees. Bring torso upright, extend arms. Hold for five deep breaths. [warrior 2, *virabhadrasana II*]

e. Extend torso over bent leg. Place left forearm on thigh, palm up. Place back hand on hip, shoulder back. Turn chest to sky. Look beyond top shoulder. Hold for five breaths. [extended side angle, *utthita parsvakonasana*]

f. Root down through legs. Then inhale, come up, straighten front leg.

g. Exhale, extend spine over front leg. Keeping legs strong, rest left arm lightly on shin. Inhale, turn torso up, look up. Extend arms out from heart. Hold for five breaths. [triangle pose, *trikonasana*]

h. Root down through the legs. Inhale, come up. Turn front foot in parallel to back foot.

i. Exhale, hands to hips, fold down. Fingertips in line with toes. Neck long. Hold for five breaths. [wide-legged forward bend, *prasarita padottanasana*]

j. Root down through legs. Inhale, hands on hips, come up.

k. Turn right foot out to back of mat. Inhale, repeat warrior 2. Hold for five breaths.

l. Exhale into extended side angle. Hold for five breaths.

m. Inhale, come up, straighten legs as before. Exhale into triangle pose. Hold for five breaths.

n. Exhale, hands to floor. Come into low lunge.

o. Step left foot up to meet the right for chair pose at the back of the mat. Hold for five breaths.

p. Exhale, root down through legs, stand tall. Hands in prayer in front of heart.

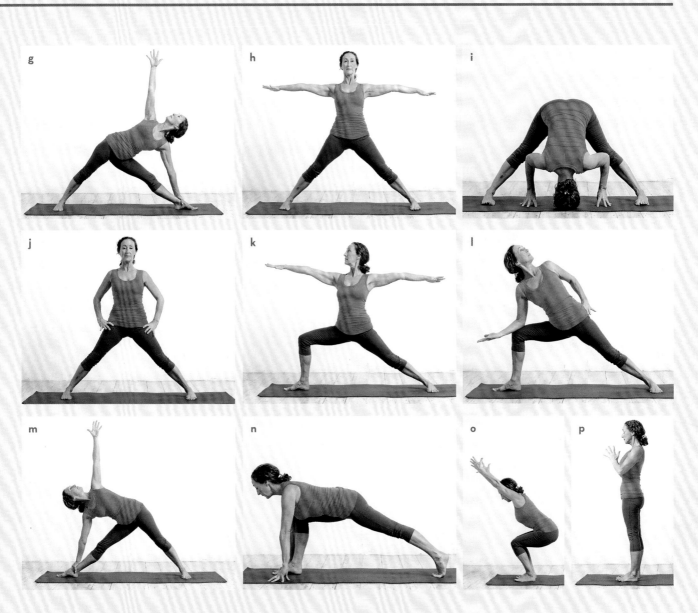

g h i

j k l

m n o p

RELAXATION 13. CENTRING

ujjayi breath meditation in hero pose

a. From kneeling sit back on heels, or with block or cushion between heels. Feel pelvis grounding, spine rising. Rest right palm on left, both face up, in your lap. Eyes closed, take *ujjayi* breathing for a couple of minutes. [hero pose, *virasana*]

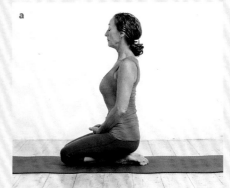

a

midday sequence – decompressing, stretching + rebalancing

BY BRIDGET WOODS-KRAMER

FOCUS: This sequence calms the mind and brings you back to a steady place at your centre. It has been designed so that it can be done in a lunch break at the office – no mat is required, just a chair and a wall.

FLOW: We begin by releasing tension in arms and shoulders caused by time spent sitting at a desk and using a computer. We move on to stretching the front of the legs, which can shorten the more time we spend in chairs. We open and strengthen hands and wrists as well as reversing the blood flow with a challenging yet brain-boosting half handstand. The sequence ends with a relaxation and breathing practice to calm the nervous system to rebalance you for the afternoon ahead.

YOU WILL NEED: A chair (non-swivel), some books or a block, a wall.

For a shorter ten-minute practice do:
1) Warm-up
4) Brain Boost
5) Strong Legs, Open Heart

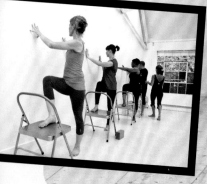

you can also follow this sequence on the DVD

1. WARM-UP

shoulder opener at wall

a. Stand 30cm (1ft) from wall side-on. Extend arm nearest the wall up and back. Step the leg furthest from the wall forwards to a gentle lunge. Keep head (top) of arm bone back, hips square. Keep shoulder blade on back. Hold for five breaths.

Repeat on other side.

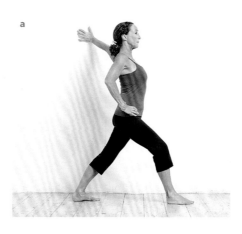

2. DECOMPRESSING THE SPINE, ENERGISING THE LEGS

a) half forward bend, b) wide-legged forward bend, c) twisting wide-legged forward bend, d) extended side angle

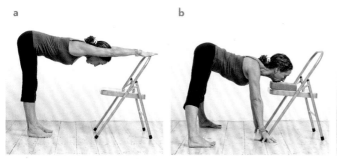
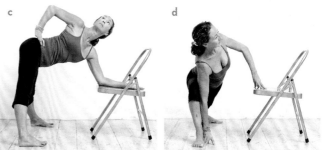

a. Stand about 0.5 metre (2ft) in front of chair. Take feet hip-width apart, rest palms on chair back. Step back until back is flat, feet below hips. Head of arm bones back, shoulder blades on back. Soften heart towards floor without dropping head. Hold for five breaths.

b. Step feet wide, parallel and in line with hips. Bring fingertips to floor under shoulders. Rest chin on chair seat; add books or block if needed. Head of arm bones back as before. Soften between shoulder blades. Hold for five breaths.

c. Keep legs wide, draw chair closer. Rest forearms and palms on seat. Place right hand on right hip. Twist to the right; chest turns to sky. Keep hips square to chair. Look up and hold for five breaths. *Repeat* **c**, *twisting to other side.*

d. Legs still wide, rest left hand on seat. Turn right foot out 90 degrees, bend right knee. Take right fingertips to floor inside foot. Root down from pelvis into back foot. Knee stays over ankle, chest turns to sky; look up. Hold for five breaths. *Repeat* **d**, *bending left knee to do other side.*

3. FOCUSING

b) dancer preparation, c) full dancer pose

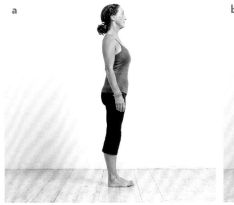
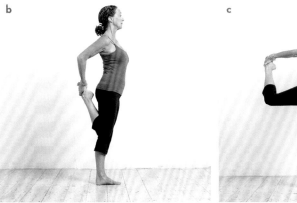

a. Begin in mountain pose. Feet hip-width apart and parallel. Arms by your sides.

b. Find a focus point at eye level. Shift weight to left leg. Place left hand on left hip. Take top of right foot in right hand, draw it towards bottom. Lengthen tailbone down and spine up. Hold balance for five breaths.

c. Raise foot behind you, pressing into hand. Root down from sit bones into your standing leg. Come forwards into bow shape (as above). Raise opposite arm for counterbalance, placing hand on wall in front for support if needed. Hold for five breaths. [dancer, *natarajasana*] *Repeat **b** and **c** on other leg.*

4. BRAIN BOOST

d) half handstand at the wall, f) child's pose

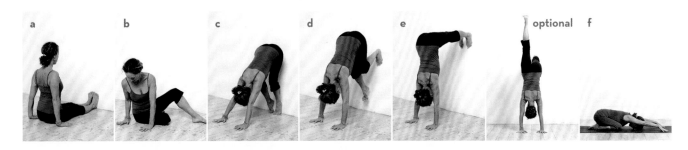

a. Sit with feet against wall as shown, hands by hips as a marker.

b. Turn around, place hands where hips were.

c. Take bent-legged downward dog, heels on wall.

d. Walk bent legs up wall, no higher than hip level. Keep arms super-strong and straight. Root from your sit bones into wall to avoid arching back.

e. Once feet reach hip height, straighten legs. Resist temptation to move hands further away from wall. Hold for five breaths.

OPTIONAL CHALLENGE:
Raise alternate legs vertically.

f. Rest in child's pose: knees wide, sit on heels. Stay until pulse returns to normal.

5. STRONG LEGS, OPEN HEART

a) chair twist at the wall, b) triangle pose, c) revolved triangle both at wall

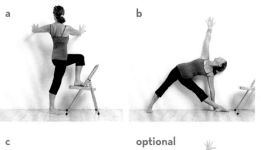

a

b

c

optional

a. Take chair side-on to wall as shown, stand in front of seat. Place foot closest to wall on seat. Twisting from the lower belly, bring hands to wall at shoulder height, chest broad. Lengthen through bent leg, keeping hips square to chair. Hold for five breaths. *Repeat other side*

b. Stand with back to wall, heels a few centimetres away. Step legs wide, turn left foot and thigh out parallel to wall. Root down through legs, inhale, lengthen spine. Exhale, extend left fingertips to right shin, right arm vertical. Lean shoulders, back of head and buttocks on wall. Look at top hand, spine long. Hold for five breaths.

Repeat on other side

c. Begin as for triangle **(b)**, heels now 15cm (6in) from wall. Turn left foot out, just in front of chair. Pivot on ball of back foot, unplug heel. Square hips to chair, hinge from hips, extend spine to chair. With straight legs, place right forearm on seat. Take left heel down if possible. Twist chest towards wall, left hand on wall. Keep spine long, not rounding. Hold for five breaths [revolved triangle, *parivrtta trikonasana*]. *Repeat on other side*

OPTIONAL CHALLENGE:
Right hand on floor inside left foot.

6. OPENING SHOULDERS, FREEING THE BREATH

a) bridge, b) eye of the needle

a (i)

a (ii)

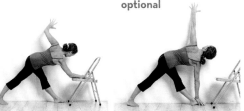

b

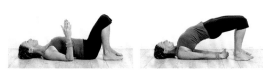

a (i). Lie with knees bent, feet parallel and below knees. Press elbows and shoulders to floor, hands parallel, fingers point up.

a (ii). Breathe in and lift chest off floor. Lift your hips as high as you can. Lengthen tailbone towards knees. Don't pull shoulders away from ears as it will flatten your neck. Clasp hands

together under back. Hold for five breaths. [bridge, *setu bandha sarvangasana*]

b. Lower buttocks to floor, cross right ankle, foot flexed, over left thigh. Draw left knee to chest with hands or belt. Keep head and shoulders on floor. Hold for five breaths. Change cross of legs and repeat. [eye of the needle]

RELAXATION 7. CENTRING

a) easy cross-legged relaxation with chair,
b) alternate nostril breathing

a

b

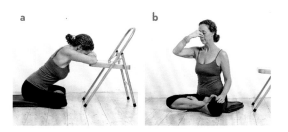

a. Sit cross-legged in front of chair. Make a pillow with your hands on chair to support your forehead. Let the mind become quiet for a couple of minutes with the breath.

b. Alternate nostril breathing. If time, spend three minutes breathing here, eyes closed. For more detailed instruction, see page 168. [alternate nostril breathing, *nadi shodana*] *Repeat approx. 20 rounds. End on exhale on left.*

evening sequence – grounding + relaxing

BY BRIDGET WOODS-KRAMER

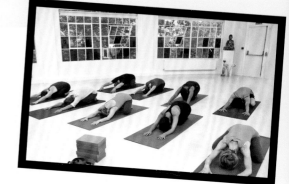

you can also follow this sequence on the DVD

FOCUS: This sequence of floor poses relaxes you and can be particularly beneficial in grounding you at the end of the day.

FLOW: Forward bends calm the nervous system, twists bring mobility to the spine. Seated poses such as pigeon and firelog release hips and improve circulation in the hips, pelvis and lower back – areas which may be tight after long hours spent sitting on a chair or in the car. The sequence finishes with a relaxing inversion, legs-up-the-wall pose and final relaxation (*savasana*).

If you have any knee pain follow the 'knee issues' options for sequence 2. Remember to turn the thighs in manually in all seated poses (see page 135) to ground the sitbones before you extend.

YOU WILL NEED: A cushion or foam block, a large towel or blanket, and a strap if you have tight hamstrings.

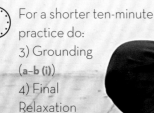 For a shorter ten-minute practice do:
3) Grounding
(a–b (i))
4) Final
Relaxation

1. WARM-UPS

a) child's pose, b) downward facing dog, c) three-legged dog,
e) lunge with twisting backbend

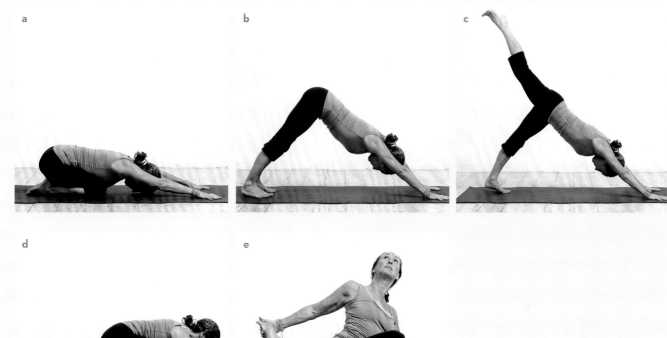

a

b

c

d

e

a. Sit on heels, feet together, knees apart. Lengthen spine, take forehead to floor. Stretch arms out in front and breathe deeply for a minute or two.

b. Inhale to all fours, tuck toes under. Lift sitbones to sky, press thighs back. Straighten your legs if possible for downward facing dog.

c. Inhale, raise right leg behind you, lifting inner thigh and inner heel. Top of left thigh moves back, hips squared.

d. Step right foot between hands to lunge. Front knee stays over ankle.

e. Drop left knee to floor. Come on to fingertips. Bend back leg towards bottom. With right hand reach for the foot (little-toe side). Take a strap around foot if necessary. Scoop tailbone down, lengthen spine, open chest to sky. Fix gaze on non-moving point. Hold for five breaths.

Repeat from **b** *(downward facing dog), raising the left leg this time at* **c** *and stepping it forwards to work the other side of the body.*

2. FLOOR SEQUENCE: OPENING HIPS AND SHOULDERS

*a) downward facing dog, b) three-legged dog, c) pigeon, d) heron, e) firelog,
f) cow face pose, g) half lord of the fishes pose*

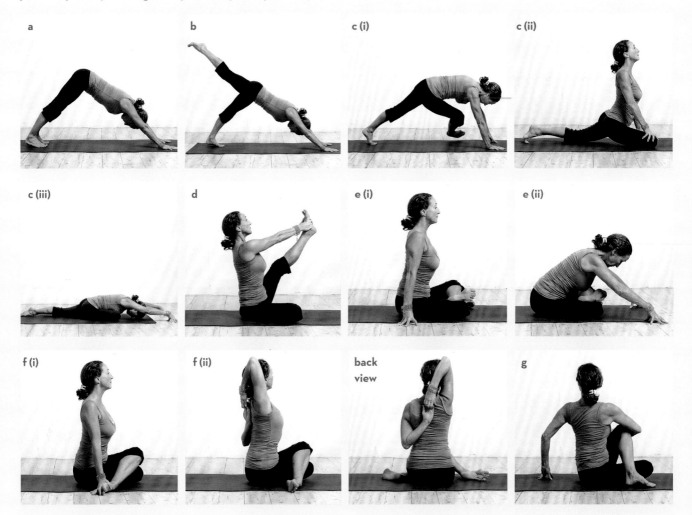

a. Begin in downward facing dog.

b. Inhale, raise right leg. Lift with inner heel and inner thigh. Keep top of left thigh moving back.

*If you have knee issues, now continue sequence from **c** on facing page*

c (i). Bend right leg and bring knee to floor behind right wrist. Take foot across mat, towards left hand.

c (ii). Square pelvis and hips to front of mat. Scoop tailbone down, lengthen through spine, lift the heart. Extend through back leg, toes tucked. Rest fingertips on floor alongside hips. (Support right buttock with cushion if needed). Hold for five breaths.

c (iii). Bow forwards, lengthen through spine. Forehead to floor. Press fingertips down, lift elbows and armpits away from floor. Melt the heart towards floor, toes pointed now. Stay here for five breaths. [one-legged king pigeon prep, *eka pada rajakapotasana* prep]

d. From pigeon walk your hands back in. Leaning to right, bring left leg out in front. Hold sides of foot or shin and stretch leg towards straight. Root down, lengthen up through spine, lift heart, shoulders back. Sit on block if your lower back is rounding. Hold for five breaths. [heron, *krounchasana*]

e (i). Bend left leg, place ankle on top of right thigh. Flex both feet, shins should now be stacked on top of each other.

e (ii). Bow forwards. Hold for five breaths. [firelog, *agnistambhasana*]

f (i). Crossing the legs deeper now, stack left knee on right at your midline. [cow face pose, *gomukhasana*]

f (ii). Inhale and stretch right arm to sky alongside ear, bend elbow so fingertips touch spine. Extend left arm to side, bend elbow and sweep arm behind back. Clasp fingers behind back. Shrug shoulders back, draw ribs in. If hands don't touch, use a strap. Press head into top arm. Hold for five breaths.

g. Release hands, bring left foot flat on floor outside right knee. Inhale, lengthen spine, exhale, turning to left, hook right elbow around outside of knee. Press thigh to left to deepen twist in lower belly. Left fingertips on floor behind you. Twist here for five breaths. [half lord of the fishes pose, *ardha matsyendrasana*]

Repeat sequence 2 on other side, this time raising left leg behind you, and doing all poses on other side of body.

FLOOR SEQUENCE VARIATIONS FOR THOSE WITH KNEE ISSUES

c (i)
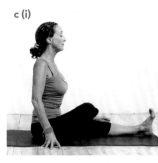

c (ii)

d
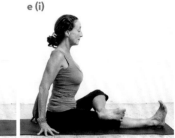

e (i)

e (ii)
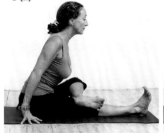

f (i)
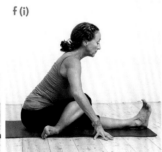

f (ii)

g
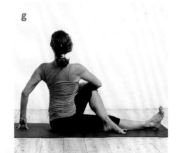

c (i). Pigeon alternative
Sit with hands alongside buttocks, legs out straight. Place right ankle on left thigh, flex feet.

(ii). Take fingertips behind you, draw left leg towards buttocks. Lengthen through spine. Lift heart towards shin. Take five breaths.

d. Heron
Extend both legs again. Bend right leg in, then take sides of left foot or shin in both hands and stretch leg towards straight.

Root down, lengthen up through spine, lift heart, shoulders back. Sit on block if your lower back is rounding, and use strap if needed.Hold for five breaths and release leg.

e (i). Firelog alternative
Straighten both legs again. Now bend left leg, place ankle on top of right thigh. Keep right leg straight, flex both feet.

e (ii). Bow forwards for five breaths. Optional: take hands in front.

f (i). Cow face pose alternative
Stack the knees a little deeper, bringing left knee on top of right at your midline. Take fingertips in front of you, extend spine. Hold for five breaths.

f (ii). Come up. Leaving legs as they are, inhale, stretch right arm to sky alongside ear. Bend elbow so fingertips touch spine, extend left arm to side, bend elbow and sweep arm behind back. Clasp fingers behind back, shrug shoulders back, draw ribs in. If hands don't touch, use a

strap. Press head into top arm. Hold for five breaths.

g. Half lord of the fishes pose alternative
Release hands, bring left foot flat on floor outside right knee. Inhale, lengthen spine, exhale, turning to left, hook right elbow around knee. Press thigh to left to deepen twist in lower belly. Left fingertips on floor behind you. Twist here for five breaths

Repeat sequence 2 on other side, this time raising left leg behind you.

3. GROUNDING

a) head-to-knee pose, b) wide angle seated forward bend with variations,
c) bound angle pose

a (i)   **a (ii)**   **b (i)**

b (ii)   **b (iii)**   **c**

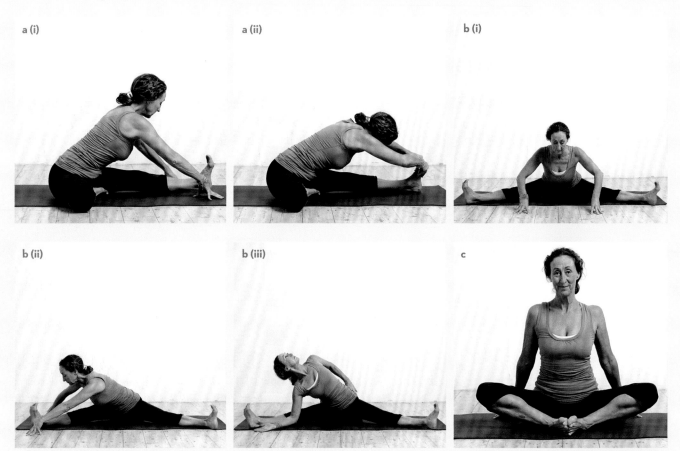

a (i). Sit with legs extended together in front, grounding the sitbones. Bend right leg, open knee out to side.

a (ii). Inhale, lengthen spine, exhale, turn and bow forwards over straight leg. Stay here for five breaths, keeping straight leg grounded, both feet flexed. Inhale, come up. Repeat on other side. [head-to-knee pose, *janu sirsasana*]

b (i). Spread legs wide, ground thighs, knees and feet face up. Sit on the edge of a cushion if your lower back is rounding. Inhale, lengthen spine, exhale, extend forward from hips. Rest fingertips on floor in front, chest broad. Hold for five to ten breaths. Inhale, come up. [wide angle seated forward bend, *upavistha konasana*]

b (ii). Turn belly, ribs and chest to right thigh. Keep thighs and pelvis grounded, feet flexed, as you extend spine over right leg. Hold for five breaths.

b (iii). Turn belly, ribs and chest to left, place right forearm, hand palm up, inside right shin. Place left hand on left hip. Shrug left shoulder back. Open heart to sky. Hold for five breaths.

*Repeat **b (ii)** and **b (iii)** on left side.*

c. Draw heels in towards groin, soles of feet together. Press little toes down into the floor, feel tops of thighs becoming heavier. Lengthen tailbone down, feel the lift in lower belly. Point fingertips backwards on floor behind buttocks, chest broad. Keeping the hands where they are, lengthen spine and bow forwards. Stay five to ten breaths. [bound angle pose, *baddha konasana*]

4. FINAL RELAXATION SEQUENCE

a) legs-up-the-wall pose with breathing exercise, b) left-nostril breathing, c) corpse pose

a   optional   b

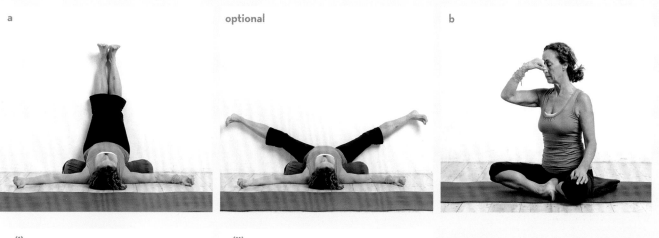

c (i)   c (ii)

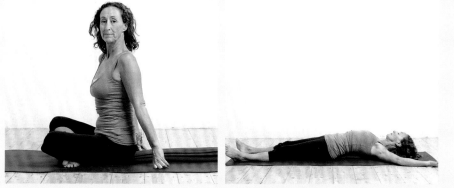

a. At the wall curl up on your side, lying 90 degrees to the wall, bottom and toes touching the wall. Roll on to back, swing legs up the wall. Keep pelvis grounded and buttocks as close to wall as possible. Place cushion (if you have one) under waistline, keep curve in lower back.

Bring hands to belly – breathe here for five breaths. Take hands to ribcage – breathe here for five breaths. Take hands to upper chest – breathe here for five breaths. Optional: take legs wide if preferred. [legs-up-the-wall pose, *viparita karani*]

b. (If short of time go straight to **c**) Sit tall, cross-legged on cushion, shoulders back. Block right nostril with right thumb. Breathe in through left nostril, close it with your ring finger, release thumb and exhale through right nostril. Repeat, inhaling through the left, exhaling right. Continue this cooling breath for three minutes. [left-nostril breathing, *chandra bhedana*]

c. If you have a towel, concertina-fold it lengthways as shown and make a pleat for the neck. Lie down, arms away from the body, palms up. Allow feet to drop outwards. Let the lips part gently, eyes closed. Relax here for five minutes (option, use an eye bag). Roll to one side to come up. [corpse pose, *savasana*]

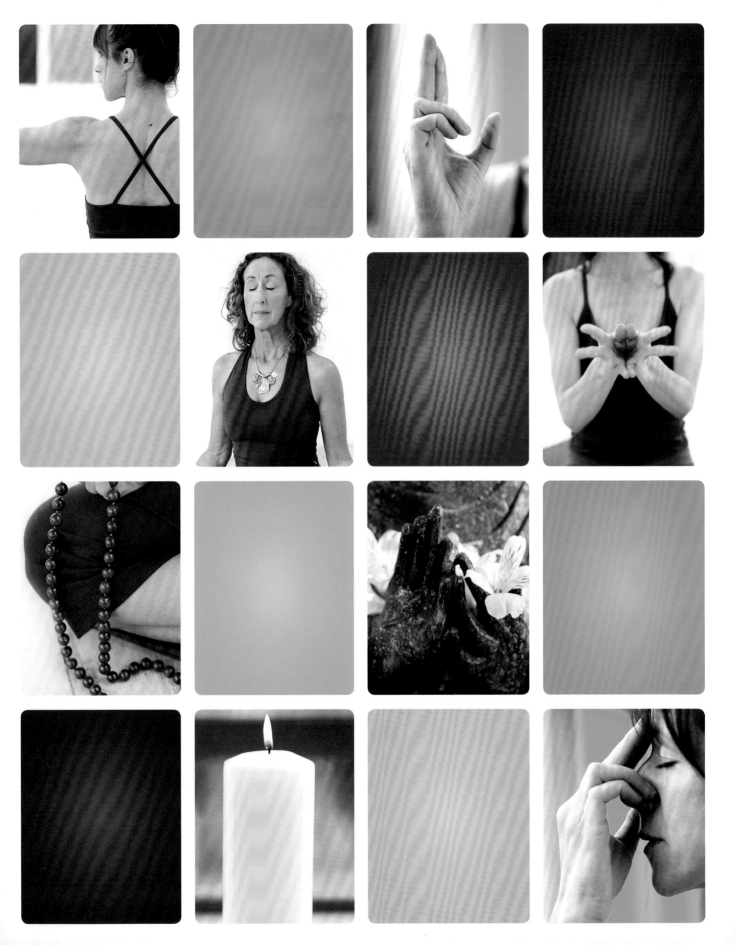

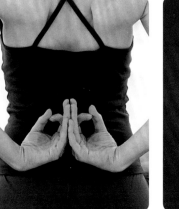
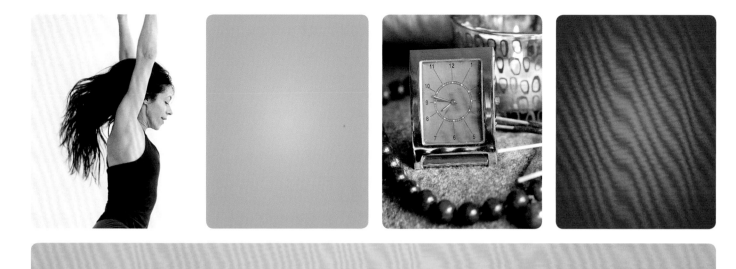

going deeper

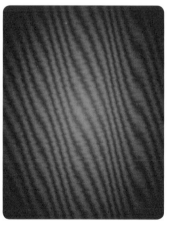
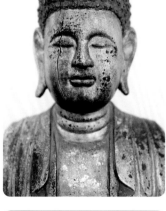
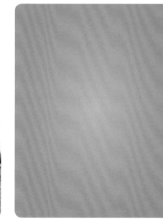
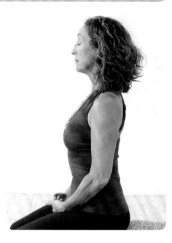

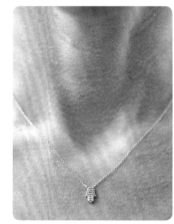
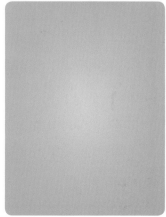

energy

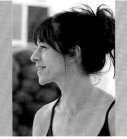

Wouldn't it be great to have more energy – or to bring the energy we have into balance so that we feel calmer and more joyful more often? Yoga recognises that we have a system of energy pathways and that we can work with it to improve how we feel. Here's how...
BY JEAN HALL

One of the first things we notice when we get up in the morning is how much energy we have – or maybe how much we lack. Some days we can spring out of bed rested and ready to take on the world, but at other times it's only an extra shot in our morning coffee or our responsibilities to others that get us going. On the other hand, if we are overloaded and overstimulated, we rush around from one task to the next without sufficient focus to see anything through. Either way, our energy is out of balance.

Becoming more centred helps cultivate clarity in our lives and can help us meet the day with joy and vitality. Directing our energy flow in an optimal way is a major step on that path.

Western science is also coming around to the idea of energy pathways, following research validating the idea that energy channels (meridians in Chinese medicine, or *nadis* in the yoga system) are located in our connective tissue.[1]

In yoga energy is known as *prana* – the universal life force that flows through us all. We can live for periods without food, water or even breath. However, without *prana* life stops. When *prana* is balanced and flowing freely to every part of our body, we feel comfortable in our own skin, calm, happy and energised – that post-yoga feeling, in fact.

But when life's stresses get in the way, *prana* can become imbalanced, deficient or stuck. Through yoga we rebalance and refresh *prana*, making us feel more vital and able to cope. This is why, when we practise yoga, we feel its effects on more than just a physical level – we are working with the very essence of life.

When we start practising yoga we begin with the physical body, because it is the most tangible aspect of our being. Yoga poses open the body up to the process of structural alignment. Our system starts to be articulated, massaged, stretched and oxygenated. Our body begins to feel measurably better – and we can start to enjoy our physicality again. Our organs function better through increased blood supply and the nervous system is calmed. The endocrine system is balanced, helping reduce the level of stress hormones. If we are less stressed, our sleep and mood may improve, which gives us more get-up-and-go.

Over time, we also learn to move our body with the breath, and this helps to release tension that can hold us in fixed patterns both physically and emotionally. By letting go of tension we liberate energy within the body; we breathe more fully and are able to feel the life and vitality within us.

And once we are more open, alive and aware, we are more able to respond to our natural patterning – taking heed of the times when we need to rest, eat and play. This is where yoga starts to go beyond the physical, connecting us to our inner wisdom. The key that links our physical body to our inner wisdom is the breath.

Our body begins to feel measurably better – and we can start to enjoy our physicality again.

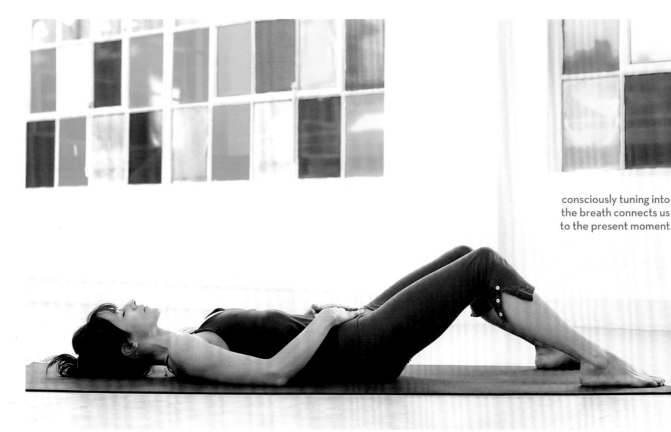

consciously tuning into
the breath connects us
to the present moment

BETTER BREATH, GREATER ENERGY

The breath is our life companion, but because it happens automatically we are rarely aware of it. Yet it is one of the most effective tools that we have for balancing the mind and nourishing the body. If we relax the breath and let it find its full and natural flow, we can lower the heart rate and soothe the nervous system. It is a powerful anchor for our mind and heart, especially when we are feeling distracted, caught up or confused. Consciously tuning in to the breath connects us to the present moment (after all, we can't breathe in the past or the future) and to our inner body, our *prana*.

Try this: Conscious breath

This exercise softly accentuates the qualities of the inhale and exhale and helps dismantle stuck breathing patterns that may have come about through trauma, illness or general day-to-day stresses and strains.
— Lie down on your back and rest your hands on your belly, as pictured above.

— Relax your body fully, feeling it soften into the floor.
— First, notice your breath without trying to change it.
— Is it short or long, shallow or deep, easy or tense?
— Now, slowly take a deep breath in through the nose until you are full. Pause here briefly.
— Now sigh your breath out fully through your mouth.
— Do this a few times to clear your lungs and your mind, and then allow your breath to return to an easy flow in and out of the nose.

Try this: Four-part breathing

The breath doesn't just consist of an inhale and exhale; it has four parts, which include the subtle pauses between the in-breath and the out-breath. Try this exercise to cultivate a fuller breath cycle:
— Lie down on your back and let your whole body relax. Inhale slowly through your nose. Feel your breath pouring into your lower lungs and abdominal area, gradually rising up to fill the upper lungs and chest.
— At the top of the in-breath notice a soft pause, as if you were going over the brow of a hill.

— As you exhale through your nose, feel your lungs emptying. Notice how the energy descends and your body releases in the floor.

— Once the out-breath is complete, feel the natural pause that follows and briefly relax into that complete passivity, emptiness and calm.

— Repeat this breathing for a minute or two, keeping the breath soft, making sure that there's no strain or pressure in the head at the top of the inhale, and that your exhale doesn't leave you gasping for the next breath. Enjoy the easy flowing rhythm and gentle pauses of nothingness.

THE NADIS – ENERGY CHANNELS

It is said that there are 72,000 energy channels called *nadis* (rivers) in the body. The most important is the *sushumna nadi* (gracious channel) which runs along the spine. Also key are *ida nadi*, the 'left-flowing' channel, representing moon and feminine energy, and *pingala nadi*, the 'right flowing' channel, which symbolises sun energy and is associated with masculine qualities. These three *nadis* originate at the base of the pelvis (*muladhara* chakra, see page 172). *Sushumna* flows centrally through the body to the crown of the head, while *ida* and *pingala* converge with *sushumna* and end their journey at the eyebrow centre (*ajna* chakra).

THE FIVE VAYUS, OR 'WINDS', OF PRANA

Prana travels through *nadis*, but is also drawn through our body in currents called *vayus* or 'winds'. The two most important *vayus* are *prana vayu*, an upward-moving energy, predominantly carried on the inhalation, and *apana vayu*, downward-moving energy, which is felt as we exhale.

Both of these energies are fundamental to our life; we need *prana vayu* to grow, lift and open, while *apana vayu* keeps us grounded and strong, and helps us with the letting-go both physically (elimination of waste) and emotionally. There are three other *vayus* (*samana*, *udana* and *vyana*) which move *prana* from side to side, in a spiralling motion through the limbs and circuiting the whole body, respectively. These *vayus* are present in us at all times but we can feel their profound momentum when we breathe. In our yoga practice we can experience these currents too. If we are mindful of the breath on the mat we can feel how every inhalation inspires an expanding, upward movement and every exhalation allows us to deepen and ground. *Asana* practice teaches us how to move in harmony with the breath – and *prana*. When we work with the natural flow of our *prana*, we are present in the flow of life. When we breathe in fully with absolute awareness, and breathe out completely, we find that we are better able to take on life's challenges and even blessings, and to let go of the situations and stresses that can limit our growth.

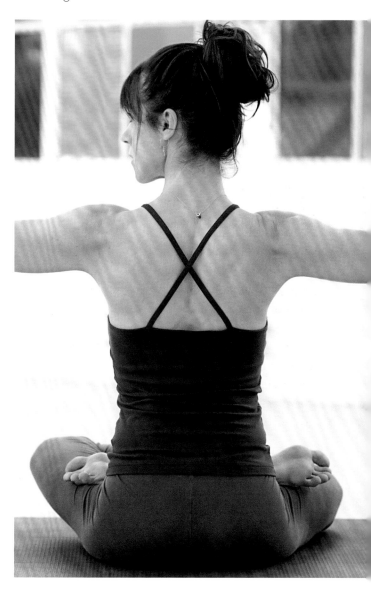

yoga breathing – pranayama

Pranayama, or 'expanding the breath', is an ancient discipline described in *The Yoga Sutras* as one of the eight limbs (or elements) of yoga (see page 18). *Pranayama* keeps the *nadis* clear and our energy circulating in an optimal way.

Breathing steadily and with awareness through the nose brings more *prana* into the body through *ida* and *pingala nadis*.

There are many *pranayama* exercises involving different patterns of inhalation, exhalation and retention (i.e. holding the breath in or out).

If done well, *pranayama* can increase lung capacity, oxygenate the blood, lead to a healthy, strong nervous system – and, so say the yogic texts, the release of the great *prana*, the *kundalini shakti*. If done badly, however, *pranayama* can deplete our energy and lead to mental disturbance (remember, we are working with vital life force). BKS Iyengar warns that *pranayama* exercises need to be extremely precise and attempted only when the yoga *asanas* have been mastered.[2] Some *pranayama* exercises, especially those involving breath retention, are contra-indicated for conditions such as high blood pressure and pregnancy. For this reason *pranayama* should be practised only under the expert guidance of an experienced teacher.

The breathing exercises given here are simple and safe and focus on deepening and connecting with the inhale and exhale.

Ujjayi breath

This is often practised throughout *asana* class, especially in dynamic styles. *Ujjayi* breath is soft and audible – like the sound of a distant ocean – and is a tool for focusing the mind. Because we can hear it, it makes it easier to synchronise our movements to the breath. In this way we can use the natural movement of the breath to support our movement, flowing with it. *Ujjayi* has an even, steady quality – the inhale and exhale are the same length – and helps to cultivate clarity of mind. For this reason, it can also be practised seated as a mindfulness meditation. *Ujjayi* translates as 'victorious' or 'triumphant' as it is believed to bring about success on the spiritual path.

How to do it:

Sit or lie comfortably. Close your eyes and shine awareness into your breath, allowing it to flow naturally. As your breath steadies, imagine you have a nostril in the front of your throat. Keeping your mouth closed, inhale and imagine the breath drawing in through that 'throat nostril', and then drawing out again the same way on the exhale. A subtle contraction will occur at the glottis (the vocal cord folds and the space in between them) in the same way as when you whisper. It creates a soft resonance, making the gentle sound 'so' as you inhale, and '*hum*' as you breathe out. *So-hum* is also a Sanskrit mantra meaning 'I am that' ('that' meaning 'oneness' or 'absolute creation').

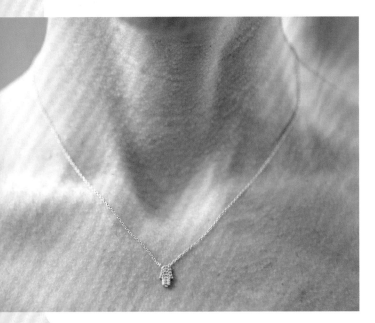

for *ujjayi* breath, imagine you have a nostril at the front of your throat

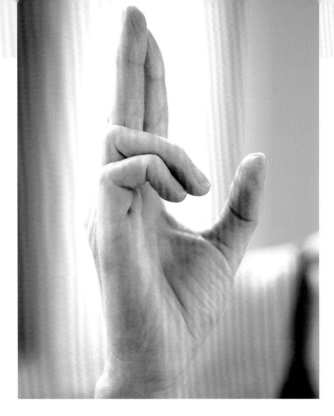

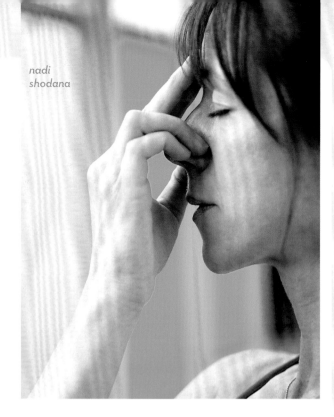

*nadi
shodana*

Nadi shodana: 'channel cleansing' breath

Here, we breathe alternately through the left and right nostrils. *Nadi shodana*, sometimes called alternate nostril breathing, calms the mind, helping to harmonise the in- and out-breaths and to balance the nervous system. Try it for a few minutes whenever you are feeling out of balance.

How to do it:

Sit comfortably, either on a chair or cross-legged on a cushion, with your back relaxed but straight. Support your back against a wall if this is uncomfortable. Close your eyes and shine awareness into your breath, allowing it to flow naturally. Take your right hand and curl your little finger and ring finger in to your palm. Extend your index and middle fingers and lightly place them between your eyebrows. Rest your thumb on your right nostril and your curled ring finger on your left nostril. Keep these fingers in contact with your nose throughout the practice, using them as valves to increase and decrease the flow of air through each nostril. To begin, close your right nostril with your thumb and gently inhale through your left for three to

four counts. Softly pinch both nostrils shut for a moment and then release your thumb and exhale fully through your right nostril for four. Inhale through your right nostril for three to four counts. Softly pinch both nostrils shut for a moment and then release your ring finger and exhale through your left nostril for four. Now inhale slowly through your left nostril for three to four counts and continue with this pattern, repeating another 18 times or so.

'Sending' your breath

Your teacher may ask you to 'send your breath' to an area of tightness or discomfort – but what do they mean? What you are being asked to do is shine the light of your awareness to those areas. If you find the idea difficult to grasp, try visualising your breath as a colour. As you breathe in, see the colour flooding that area. Effectively, what we are doing is directing *prana* with our awareness. It is said that where our awareness goes, *prana* flows.

As we are working on a subtle level, directing *prana* is a quiet, mindful practice, a deep sensing and awakening within the body.

energy locks – the bandhas

Prana can seep out from our extremities and facial features: for example, our hands, fingers, feet, toes, eyes, pelvis or even through our thought waves. This is where our *bandhas* – our internal energy locks – come in. *Bandhas* not only seal *prana* in, they also concentrate its energy in order to redirect it. They have been likened to the damming of a river. Once the dam is opened (i.e. the bandhas have been released after practice) energy pours into the surrounding areas or the entire body, recharging, rebalancing and relaxing us.

The primary aim of the *bandhas* is to seal off energy to certain areas and redirect it into the *sushumna nadi* (central energy channel) in order to generate spiritual awakening: *kundalini shakti*.

What's perhaps more relevant for us is that the *bandhas* produce heat in the body. And, as the principal quality of heat is purification, they play a powerful role in clearing the *nadis*, so that our energy can flow in an optimal way and we feel more vital. Each *bandha* also tones the muscles around it, promoting strength and stability, which helps minimise injury in *asana* practice.

Bandhas are arch-shaped structures found in the arches of the feet and hands, the perineal lift, the diaphragm at the abdomen, upper diaphragm at the throat, in the upper palate and the dome of the skull. We aim to have three main *bandhas* engaged throughout our practice (see below), but that doesn't mean tensing or gripping the muscles hard. They can be subtly stimulated simply by bringing awareness to these areas using the breath, especially in *ujjayi* breathing which can help to engage all three *bandhas*.

1. Mula bandha – the root lock

Situated at the perineum at *muladhara* chakra, *mula bandha* seals off the lower pelvis so that downward-flowing *prana* cannot escape. *Mula bandha* strengthens the pelvic floor, helps support the pelvic organs and functions and stimulates *muladhara* chakra to help awaken *kundalini shakti*. Mula means 'root'.
How to find it: Sit cross-legged on the edge of a cushion. Gently press the perineum down into the floor. Now lift that area up without tensing or gripping the buttocks or the sphincter muscles of the anus. Pushing down makes it easier initially to find the lifting action that is *mula bandha*.

2. Uddiyana bandha – the abdominal lock

This is found at *manipura* chakra at the navel centre. *Uddiyana* means 'upwards flying'. Lifting the diaphragm and abdominal muscles encourages *prana* to fly upwards along *sushumna nadi*. This also creates a physical lightness that can help when tackling a tricky pose as it gives an extra lift of energy and strength to body and mind. This *bandha* doesn't so much stop energy leaking, but intensifies the energy within us. Imagine the effect of holding a hosepipe and squeezing it to make the jet more powerful.
How to find it: Practise cat/cow (see page 143), rounding and arching the spine on all fours. As you round the back at the end of the out-breath, find the hollowing of your abdomen as your navel draws up towards your spine. Because *uddiyana* engages the core, it plays a vital role in protecting the lower back. It also gives support to the internal organs.

the water here shows the arch of *hasta bandha*, the hand lock

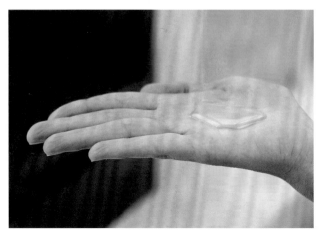

3. Jalandhara bandha – the throat lock

This is located at *vishuddhi* chakra. *Jalandhara* means 'mesh' or 'net' and catches the energy as it rises from the torso, preventing it escaping through the head.
How to find it: *Jalandhara bandha* is naturally engaged when the chin is drawn downwards to the notch at the centre of your collarbones, as in shoulder stand (right) and plough pose. It also helps cultivate *ujjayi* breathing.
Try this: Initiate a yawn, keeping your mouth closed, and then change it into an inhalation through the nose instead. Can you feel the subtle contraction in the glottis and the lower diaphragm? You may also feel a soft lift of the abdomen (*uddiyana bandha*).

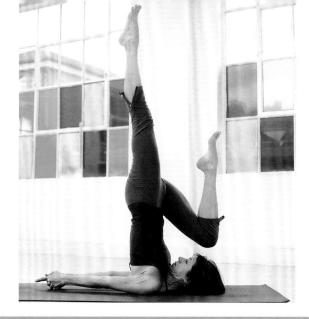

mudra – energy in a gesture

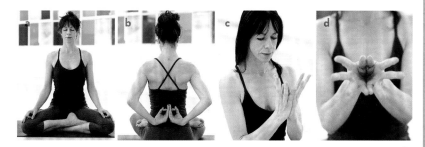

Those hand gestures that look so decorative in yoga photos and on Indian statues aren't just about aesthetics. Called *mudras* (meaning to draw forth delight), they redirect *prana* internally – in the same way that sound echoes off a wall or light bounces off a mirror. The classic hand *mudra* is *jnana mudra*, which links the thumb and index finger and creates a looped circuit of energy flowing from the brain down to the hand and back up again.

A *mudra* can also be the subtle direction of the gaze, the application of a *bandha* or a 'whole body' *mudra* using a combination of *pranayama*, *asana*, *bandha* and visualisation. *Mudras* also cultivate certain moods or attitudes and perceptions while strengthening concentration and deepening awareness. Adopting certain

body positions affects how we feel: when we stand tall and strong it helps assert a confident mood, or if we hunch over we may feel our spirit drop.
Try this: Closing your eyes can be a *mudra*. Notice how the energy and focus that radiated out through them is now being reflected back in. Feel how this natural *mudra* subtly alters your mood and awareness.

Hand mudras

These are used especially in meditation practices.
— *Jnana mudra*, the psychic gesture of knowledge practised with the palms facing down **(a)**,

helps connect us to our inner wisdom.
— *Chin mudra* uses the same loop, but is practised with the palms facing up **(b)**, and is the psychic gesture of consciousness.
— *Lotus mudra* **(c & d)** symbolises opening to the divine in our heart.

In both *jnana* and *chin mudra*, the index finger curling beneath the thumb signifies the individual self bowing to the universal soul. Becoming aware of this energetic flow leads to deep inner sensing (*pratyahara*, the fifth limb of yoga).

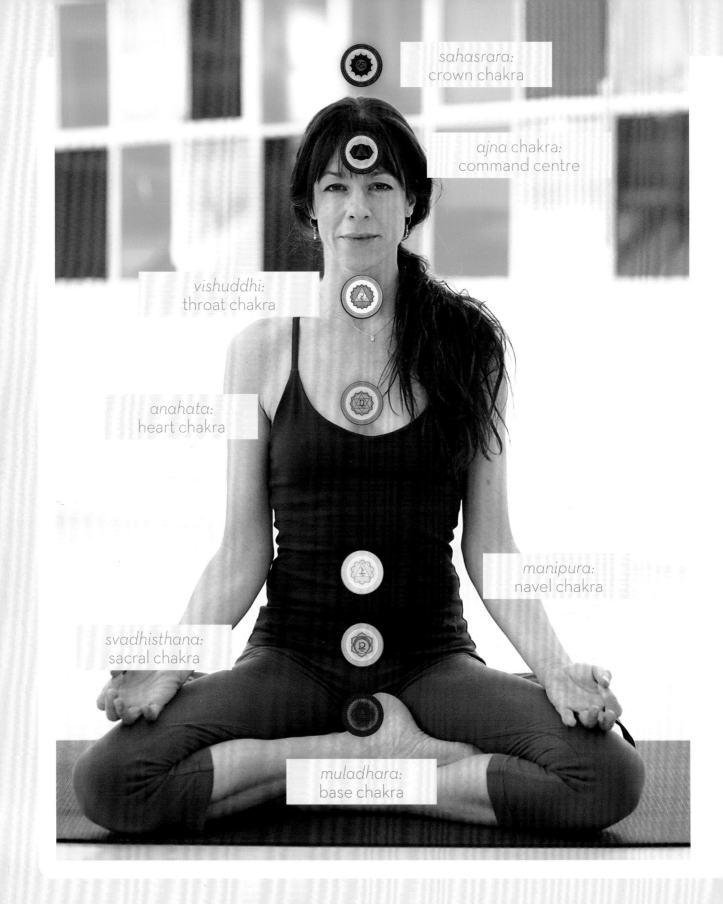

sahasrara:
crown chakra

ajna chakra:
command centre

vishuddhi:
throat chakra

anahata:
heart chakra

manipura:
navel chakra

svadhisthana:
sacral chakra

muladhara:
base chakra

the seven chakras

In yoga, we pay a great deal of attention to articulating the spine. It not only houses the main channel of our nervous and skeletal system, but also on an energetic level it is home to the most important energy channel – the *sushumna nadi*. Along *sushumna* there are said to be hubs of activity where many *nadis* converge. These are known as chakras ('wheels') – spinning vortices of energy. In Western science they correspond to nerve ganglia – clusters of nerves at the major plexuses of the body such as the solar plexus, the cervical plexus, the lumbar plexus and sacral plexus.

The chakras are like mini brains, each housing different aspects of our inner wisdom and psychological development. How open or closed our chakras are is said to affect how we feel, respond to situations and how we project ourselves.

When *prana* moves through the *sushumna nadi*, the chakras are opened and balanced. If a chakra is too open, too much light/blood/energy flows through, flooding it, and the behaviour associated with it becomes excessive. If it's too closed, not enough flows through and the associated behaviour becomes deficient. Imbalance of a chakra is also said to affect physical wellbeing. How open or closed a chakra is is thought to affect energy flow from the related plexus to the corresponding organs and glands, and so to determine how well they function.

Through conscious practice and deep continuous awareness, we can address many areas of our life through chakra work, helping to shift even long-held patterns of behaviour to create greater balance and harmony in our lives. That's not to say that working with the chakras is in any way a substitute for professional help from a therapist or doctor. But in yoga it can be used as an adjunct or support.

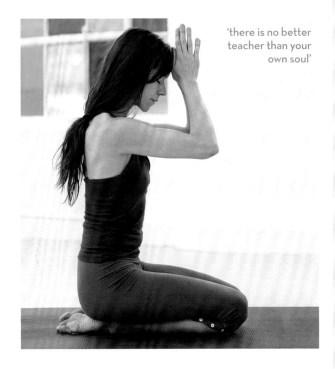

'there is no better teacher than your own soul'

TOOLS FOR BALANCING CHAKRAS

1. Yoga asana. Specific types of poses can open up specific chakras. Standing poses work *muladhara* chakra for example, while twists energise *manipura*.

2. Sound. We can also use sound – or mantra– as a way of bringing awareness to the chakras. Each chakra also has a *bija* (seed) mantra, a primordial sound that resonates deeply within the centre of each chakra, helping to unlock its energy.

3. Colour visualisation. Each chakra has a colour associated with it, which we can 'send' to that area in the same way as we 'send' our breath.

Try this: Imagine a blank screen at the location of a particular chakra, and as you breathe, see its corresponding colour pouring into that area, making it vibrant and alive. Now allow the colour to pour out, like paint dripping onto the floor.

the seven chakras in detail

Muladhara:
the base chakra

Location: the centre of the pelvic floor
Meaning: root
Centre of: basic survival needs – eating sleeping, standing, shelter, elimination
Sense: smell
Organ and gland: nose and adrenal glands
Colour: red
Bija mantra: the sound *'lam'*
Imbalance issues: weight problems, sleep issues, constipation, immune system dysfunction (e.g. arthritis), anxiety, defensiveness, victim mentality
Chakra-balancing poses: standing poses and hip-openers such as squats (e.g. *malasana*, garland pose)

Svadhisthana:
the sacral chakra

Location: between the pubic bone and navel
Meaning: 'sweetness' or 'abode of self'
Centre of: pleasure, sensuality, creativity
Sense: taste
Organ and gland: tongue and ovaries/testicles
Colour: sunset orange
Bija mantra: *'vam'*
Imbalance issues: uterine, bladder, kidney, prostate and fertility problems, decreased libido, frigidity, impotence, pleasure seeking, addiction, anhedonia (inability to feel pleasure), blocked creativity
Chakra-balancing poses: standing poses and hip-openers, such as reclining bound angle (*supta baddha konasana*)

Manipura:
the navel chakra

Location: the navel
Meaning: 'city of jewels'
Centre of: power, strength, confidence and self-esteem
Sense: vision
Organ and gland: ears and pancreas
Colour: yellow
Bija mantra: *'ram'*
Imbalance issues: diabetes, digestive problems (e.g. reflux and heart burn, ulcers, irritable bowel), domineering and controlling behaviour or lack of confidence and self-esteem
Chakra-balancing poses: *uddiyana bandha*, twists, bow pose

Anahata:
the heart chakra

Location: at the level of the heart
Meaning: 'unstruck sound'
Centre of: unconditional love, empathy and compassion
Sense: touch
Organ and gland: skin and thymus gland
Colour: green
Bija mantra: *'yam'*
Imbalance issues: circulatory and heart disease, respiratory disease, asthma, high blood pressure, oversharing or lack of empathy and compassion. As meridian lines flow from the heart through to the arms and hands, carpal tunnel, frozen shoulder and tennis elbow can be related to *anahata*.
Chakra-balancing poses: backbends and shoulder openers (e.g. *gomukhasana*)

Vishuddhi:
the throat chakra

Location: the throat
Meaning: purification
Centre of: purity and acceptance
Sense: hearing
Colour: blue
Organ and gland: ears and thyroid
Bija mantra: *'ham'*
Imbalance issues: colds, sore throat, thyroid problems, ear infections, hearing problems, being overcritical, difficulty in expressing oneself verbally or being able to discern
Chakra-balancing poses: shoulder stand, plough

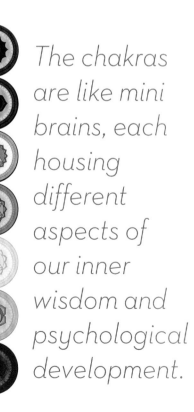

The chakras are like mini brains, each housing different aspects of our inner wisdom and psychological development.

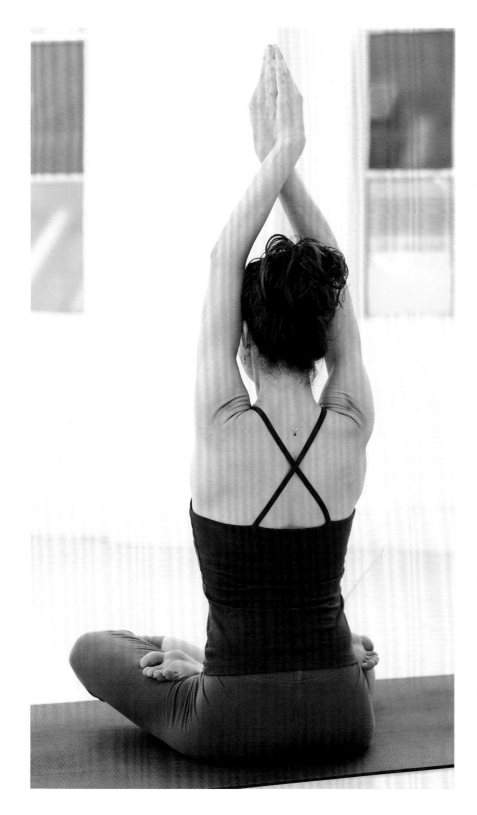

Ajna chakra: the command centre

Location: the third eye centre, between the eyebrows

Meaning: to perceive or command

Centre of: wisdom, intuition

Sense: the sixth sense – intuition

Organ and gland: psychic mind and pineal gland

Colour: violet

Bija mantra: 'sam'

Imbalance issues: headaches, visual problems, ungroundedness, being too caught up in the psychic realm, over-intellectualising, insomnia, mental disorders, inability to trust one's instincts

Chakra-balancing poses: inversions – particularly headstand

Sahasrara: the crown chakra

(Not so much a chakra but the seat of our highest consciousness and connection to all)

Location: the crown of the head

Meaning: 'thousand-fold lotus'

Centre of: highest consciousness and connection to all

Organ and gland: mind and pituitary gland

Colour: all the colours of the rainbow

Bija mantra: 'aum'

Sense: complete boundless awareness

Imbalance issues: brain imbalances (e.g. confusion, Alzheimer's), chronic exhaustion, abandonment of personal and life responsibilities, lack of embodiment and connection, hyperactive mind, anxiety, negative thinking patterns, obsessive compulsive disorders

Chakra-balancing poses: seated and/or walking meditation, *pranayama*

meditation

Meditation is at the heart of all yoga. One reason why we do physical yoga practices is so that we can sit comfortably in meditation without being distracted by a creaky body. But you don't need to have done yoga to try meditation. All you need is an interest in quieting your mind and looking inwards.
BY VICTORIA WOODHALL

More and more people are becoming interested in meditation, particularly in the past 40 years, since the Beatles and their Transcendental Meditation guru the Maharishi Mahesh Yogi brought this ancient practice to popular consciousness in the late 1960s. Science is now validating its health benefits, with studies showing its effectiveness for a range of conditions, from anxiety and insomnia to psoriasis, fibromyalgia and chronic fatigue syndrome, as well as its role in boosting disease-fighting antibodies, improving performance under stress and reducing cognitive decline in old age.

But what is meditation exactly? In a triyoga workshop with meditation teacher and yoga historian Carlos Pomeda, the group (some of whom had done meditation before, some of whom were new to the practice) was asked what they thought meditation was. They came up with this list:

- stillness
- focusing the mind on one point
- turning the mind and the senses inwards
- connecting to the Self
- being present
- calm awareness
- mindfulness
- prayer

Meditation is all of these things and more. Yet so often our days are filled with quite the reverse. We receive so much stimulation and sensory bombardment that we rarely experience sustained moments of stillness where we feel 'present' or 'in the moment' or connected to ourselves.

Sometimes we have glimpses that such stillness is possible – when we see a beautiful sunset that stops us in our tracks or when we hold our baby for the first time. For those few moments nothing else exists. We are totally in that moment without a thought. We experience something bigger than ourselves and intimately connected to ourselves – be it love, calm, or lightness, or the feeling of being exactly where we are meant to be.

While the catalyst for that feeling is external, the internal experience of centredness is of our own making. Through the practice of meditation we can train our 'mental muscles' to visit this experience more often and to keep our chattering thoughts at bay.

There's nothing mysterious about this time-honoured practice. It is not an altered state, but simply a technique of turning our attention from the outside world to our inner landscape, to a place where we are not our thoughts or feelings but where we simply witness them. It's not that we switch off entirely but that we are able to notice our thoughts with an attitude of calm awareness without becoming involved.

'It's remarkable how liberating it feels to be able to see that your thoughts are just thoughts and that they

A common misconception about meditation is that it's about making the mind go blank.

a string of beads (*mala*) is sometimes used to help count mantra repetitions are not "you" or "reality",' notes professor Jon Kabat-Zinn, a pioneer in the health applications of mindfulness meditation. The simple act of recognising this, he adds, 'can free you from the distorted reality they often create and allow for more clear-sightedness and a greater sense of manageability in your life'.[1]

It's not surprising that meditation-based practices are now being recommended by the National Institute for Health and Clinical Excellence (NICE) in the UK to help prevent people with depression from relapsing.[2]

BUT I CAN'T MAKE MY MIND GO BLANK!

A common misconception about meditation is that it's about emptying the mind completely. What we are working towards is giving less attention to our thoughts, screening them out in the same way that we use earplugs to screen out loud music.

Because meditation is ostensibly a practice of not doing, it's easy to think that it should be fairly simple to master – like walking one minute, and standing still the next. As cellular geneticist turned Buddhist monk Matthieu Ricard points out, working with the mind in order to improve it requires the same kind of sustained effort and enthusiasm that we happily give to acquiring other life skills such as learning to walk, read or write or to gain professional skills.[3] We don't mind putting in the effort because we know that in the long run these skills will benefit us, he says in his book *The Art of Meditation*. 'Working with the mind follows the same logic. How could it be subject to change without the least effort, just from wishing alone? That doesn't make any more sense than expecting to learn to play a Mozart Sonata just by occasionally doodling around on a piano.

'We expend a lot of effort to improve the external conditions of our lives, but in the end it's always the mind that creates our experience of the world and translates it into wellbeing or suffering,' he observes. 'If we transform our way of perceiving things, we transform the quality of our lives.'

How do we do this? 'By the form of mind training known as meditation,' says Ricard. As you will see from the steps below, drawn from the workshops of Carlos

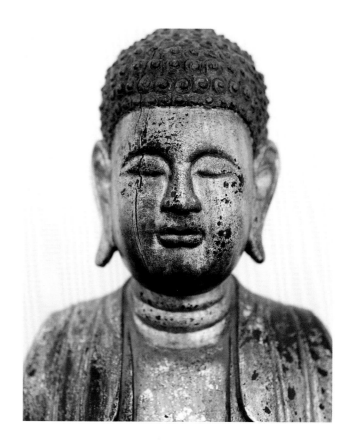

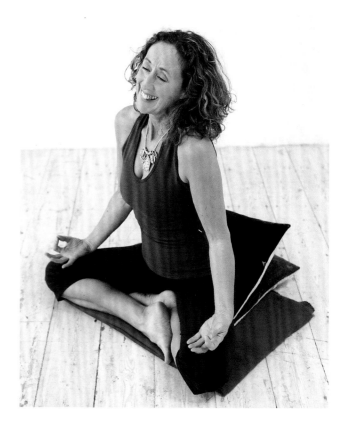

Pomeda, meditation begins actively with techniques such as scanning the body and counting the breaths, yet takes us into a very deep state. We are still aware of sounds, sensations and pulsations in the body and field of perception. But behind all this is a sense of steadiness, rootedness and calm awareness.

WHY DO WE MEDITATE?

Imagine trying to look at your reflection in a pool of water. If that water is turbulent or muddied, the image you see is of yourself distorted – if you can see anything at all. But if it is still, your true reflection shines back. *The Yoga Sutras* tell us that in the same way, only when the mind becomes truly still – unruffled by thoughts and emotions that pass across it – can we perceive our true nature.[4] Our Self.

But what is this Self? As Kabat-Zinn notes, it's not who our thoughts say we are – these are just thoughts after all. Nor is it any of the identities we project onto the outside world, be that as mother, boss, winner, loser, victim and so on. The Self – or Consciousness – is who we are in essence, when all of those layers are peeled away.

In her book *Meditation for the Love of It*[5] (recommended as further reading), meditation expert Sally Kempton explains that the Self has three essential qualities.

She writes that it is *sat* – ever present and permanently real, the thread on which the beads of our thoughts, experiences and perceptions are strung. It underlies and contains all our thoughts and experiences, but in itself is neutral and unchanging.

Second, it is *chit* – aware of itself and everything else. It is the screen on which we experience our inner and outer life as well as the part that watches the screen – our inner knower or witness.

And lastly it is *ananda*, or joyful. 'Of course this is one of the most basic teachings of yoga,' says Kempton. 'Our experiences of happiness are only possible because happiness is already inside us. It is not the other person, the beautiful scene, the film or the tiramisu that creates joy. These things may trigger it, but the joy is intrinsic to us.'[6] Think back to the last time you felt one of those moments of unexpected

connectedness. You would probably describe it more as a deep inner joy or knowing rather than something that you were able to intellectualise.

Kempton reminds us that if a successful meditation is one where we enter the Self, we have to approach each session with this as our goal.[7] Losing ourselves in thoughts, reveries, shopping lists and old arguments may be easy enough to do as we sit for meditation, but it doesn't leave us feeling satisfied or at peace.

Of all the three aspects of the Self, the one that tends to be the most easily accessible is the inner knower – the part of us that is watching our experience. Kempton suggests sitting quietly and imagining observing your body from all sides 'as if you had 360-degree awareness'. Then asking yourself, 'Who or what is witnessing my body? Who or what is witnessing my thoughts?' and, rather than answering the question verbally, 'feel the experience that arises in response to that question.' Many people, she adds, notice 'a spacious presence that often seems to be located somewhere above and behind the head'.

So while meditation begins with the mind, it can take us to a place far beyond the mind – a place of being, knowing and joy.

Now we know what the Self might be and feel like, what about the question of why we want to experience it? Quite apart from the health benefits of the practice, getting to know our Self can help rid us of our doubts and fears. Sally Kempton explains that a primary teaching of the Indian yogic traditions is that not knowing our true nature causes fears, doubts and suffering.[8] However, knowledge of the Self (via meditation) can 'burn away' these negative qualities.

Being less anxious and more confident would for most of us represent a significant improvement in our lives. Ricard adds that working with the mind can help us shift aspects of ourselves that we don't like – negative character traits that we may wrongly believe to be hardwired into our system. 'Our emotions, moods and bad character traits are merely temporary, circumstantial elements of our nature,' he explains.[9] Our core of Consciousness is neutral and unaffected by them – and once we realise this, it becomes clear that our negative character traits don't define us, and we don't have to live with them.

Meditation can also be a path towards more desirable states of mind, such as deep-felt confidence and altruistic love. In the Buddhist tradition, loving kindness meditation starts with the meditator cultivating compassion towards him- or herself, then towards those around them (including those they don't like!), and finally towards all living beings.

'Primarily,' says Ricard, 'meditation is a matter of familiarising ourselves with a clear and accurate way of seeing things and of cultivating the good qualities that remain dormant inside until we make the effort to bring them out.'[10]

While the practice itself is not always easy, in short, we meditate to try to have a nicer day, every day.

THAT'S THE THEORY, NOW FOR THE PRACTICE

How do we turn our attention inwards and keep it there without becoming distracted? The key component of meditation is our ability to concentrate – a skill that many of us use every day when we focus on a task at work, read a book, put up a shelf or play a sport. The point at which the racket hits the ball or the hammer hits the nail may be a moment of total focus where no thoughts intrude. In meditation the principle is the same. Focus and concentration, aided by techniques such as mantra, are our ways into the experience that is meditation. Practising yoga *asana* helps to hone our powers of concentration. The key to balance poses, for example, is focus – if the mind is unstable, so are we. If we move with awareness of the breath and body in real time, we are effectively practising meditation in motion.

The reality, even for experienced meditators, is that the focus gets knocked off its perch by our thoughts. It's helpful to think of meditation like a dog-training exercise. When we are newer to the practice, our mind is like a naughty puppy, jumping up at us for attention or pulling us away to chase an interesting distraction. We have to bring it to heel time and again. The puppy eventually responds to training and needs less prompting to walk by our side.

If your mind wanders, don't think that your meditation is not working. 'Our lives are so different from those of the ancient yogis who developed these techniques. They had already renounced life's stresses and in their entire lifetime would not have had to process the amount information that crosses our path in a single day,' explains Pomeda. We are trying to find calm in the midst of possibly the most overstimulated era ever and powering down is a much bigger task. 'It is very natural for memories and images to come to the surface. It's part of the mind's natural healing process,' he adds.

The key is to keep drawing the mind back to your point of focus. Even sessions where your mind feels like it will never settle are beneficial, says Pomeda. 'Just doing it is what works, not worrying about how deep you are going.'

If your mind wanders, don't think that your meditation is not working.

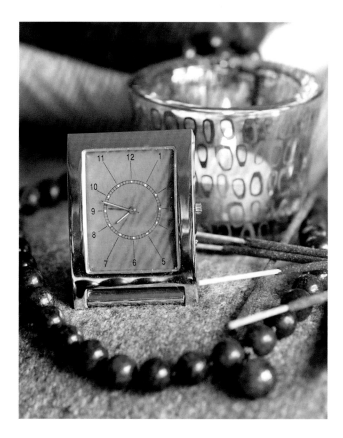

meditation – the basics

First find a time of day

Traditionally sunrise and sunset are the most sacred and powerful times for meditation. In the early morning, your mind is relatively still and your day has yet to steal your attention. An evening meditation practice helps to put your day behind you and prepare for sleep. Whatever time of day you choose, creating a habit is helpful. But if a regular time is not possible, do it whenever you can. Carlos Pomeda describes meditation as 'a muscle we need to flex every day, and one that gets better the more we train it'.

Then decide how long

Five minutes is better than nothing, but you need to sit for at least 20 minutes if you are serious about results, says Pomeda. More than 90 minutes, he adds (unless you are on retreat), brings diminishing returns. If 20 minutes is difficult at first, try setting a timer for ten and building up. With practice you will be able to programme yourself to come out of meditation after a specific time.

It is best not to meditate on a full stomach – digestion uses up energy, so you won't be getting the best out of your meditation.

Next find a space

If possible, have a dedicated place where you do nothing but meditate. The mind performs better when association is set between an action and a particular space, says Pomeda. For this reason, it's best not to meditate in bed as you may nod off. You want to be relaxed but alert. Making your space smell and look nice with inspiring pictures, symbols or candles will help cement that association.

Choose a sitting position

The original meaning of the word *asana* (which we generally use to describe a yoga posture) is 'seat'. The very first *asanas* were seated meditation postures.

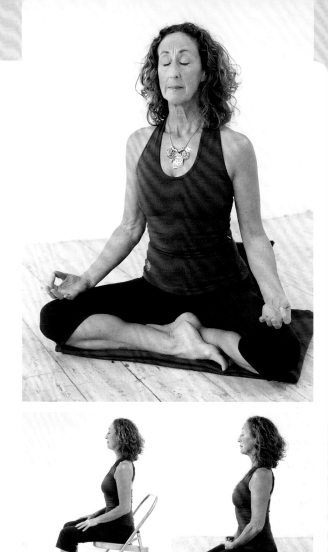

Patanjali's *Yoga Sutras* (see page 18) say that our seat should be steady and comfortable. This advice may be 2,000 years old but it's still valid today; spending time setting up your seat will improve the quality of your meditation.

Meditation *asana* can be any seated posture in which the spine is able to extend upright. Notice how much more alert you feel if you sit up straight as opposed to slumping into a chair. Use whatever blocks, blankets and bolsters you need for support so you can sit or kneel without any tension.

See over the page for some options of how to sit in meditation.

Sitting options

— **Cross-legged on the floor:** in this position you need to be able to relax your hips completely. So, unless you have very open hips, place cushions under your knees for support, sit on the edge of a block or cushion (as high up as you need for your knees to drop below your hips) and place a folded blanket underneath you so that your feet aren't squashed against a hard floor. If you need the wall for support, try coming away from it in the last five minutes and over time weaning yourself off it. If you experience pins and needles in your legs, focus on hip-openers in your yoga practice.

— **Kneeling:** sit with knees either side of a bolster placed lengthways or sit up high on blocks. Put a blanket under your knees and feet for comfort.

— **On a chair:** the ancient yogis didn't use chairs because they didn't have them. But feel free to use one. Sit with a straight spine (try not to lean into the chair back) with feet flat on the floor (use blocks or books underneath them if they don't reach).

Set up your base

If your back becomes tired in meditation, the problem is likely to be at the base – in the pelvis. Try tilting the tailbone back and seeing how your spine moves to compensate. Play with the angle of the pelvis to see where it needs to be for the spine to be upright.

Position the shoulders and hands

Hunching creates shoulder tension, so make sure the shoulders sit squarely at the top of the spine, that the shoulder blades are relaxed on the back, the upper chest is open and the neck is free. Experiment to find the most comfortable place for your hands, such as:

— Palms down on your knees (take care that this doesn't bring your shoulders forwards) or thighs.

— Palms up and, if you like, with index finger and thumb gently joined to make a circle (*chin mudra*, see page 171), the gesture of consciousness.

— In your lap, with palms face up, one over the other.

Position your head

Make sure your head is neither hanging back nor nodding forwards. It should be positioned centrally at the top of your spine, where it will feel lighter.

Scan and relax your body

Set the timer. With eyes closed, scan your body from your feet upwards, consciously relaxing each body part with the breath. As you send your mind's eye to your feet, say internally, 'My feet are relaxed.' Continue up to your calves and beyond until you have covered every part of your body, including belly, face and scalp.

Make any minor adjustments to your posture as you go, but without losing your focus.

Bring your focus to your breath

First observe the breath for a minute or so without changing it.

Then even out the breath so that the inhale and the exhale are of equal length. Slowing down and evening out the breath does the same for the mind, bringing about the mental conditions for awareness.

Don't try too hard. Just allow the breath to happen. Your breath might be deep or shallow. A shallow breath can happen when we are very relaxed as we are not drawing much oxygen to support the muscles.

Choose a technique

Once you have completed your body scan and evened out the breath, you can then simply observe the breath, or choose a meditation technique to bring your attention inwards.

Here are three suggestions: experiment with what works for you.

1. Counting the breath: This is one of the oldest techniques. Count the number of beats in your breath (for example, 'Inhale, two, three, four, five, six. Exhale, two, three, four, five, six). Most people have a count of about five or six.

2. Mantra: Repeating a Sanskrit mantra internally gives the mind something to do. But because a mantra is a sound, or combination of sounds, rather than a word that holds meaning for us, it doesn't create more activity in the mind; rather it draws us in. If you don't have a mantra given to you by a meditation teacher, then try 'Om', the universal mantra. Repeat it internally on the inhale and again on the exhale for as many times as you need to take you to a place of silence and awareness.

Some practitioners use *mala*, a string of 16, 27, 54 or 108 beads to help count the number of mantra repetitions. The larger 'guru' bead indicates the end of that round of repetitions and reminds us of our own teacher and inner teacher.

You may also like to try putting on a recording of continuous 'Om' sounds and just listening, allowing the sound to draw you inwards.

3. Visualisation: See a pure white light in the centre of your chest, at your heart, and keep your focus on this one point. If you find the visual aspect of this doesn't sit well for you, translate it into a feeling.

Explore different techniques. Trust the practice and allow it to show you what works for you. If one technique feels unnatural, try it a few more times – it may just be a question of developing a habit. If you start with a visualisation but find your mind automatically coming to the breath, use this as your focus instead.

You may feel that after a few minutes the technique is getting in the way and that you can feel quieter without it. If so, that's a sign that your meditation is working and you can let the technique go and just be.

Meditation on the go

If you have time on your hands, rather than checking your phone, try turning your attention inwards – being aware of yourself, in your body, with your breath. If you are facing a difficult issue or can't see clearly, use these moments to calm the mind, to find space between your thoughts and to come back to yourself. Being able to experience who we really are in the midst of turmoil gives us a better perspective of whatever is going on. The more we pay into the bank of calm centredness, the greater the payback in daily life.

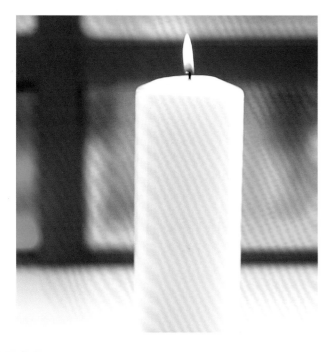

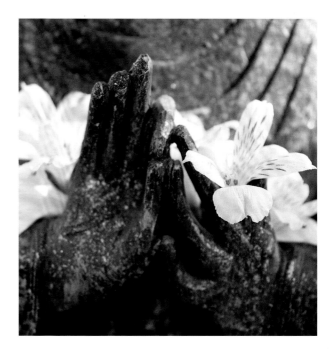

contributors

Anna Ashby

A transformational yoga meditation weekend with a friend set dancer and chorographer Anna Ashby on a new path of self-discovery – living and studying yoga at a meditation ashram in New York. It was here that she discovered the power of restorative yoga, 'for me the closest practice to meditation, which is the core practice of the yoga tradition'. She has been studying and practising yoga for more than 20 years and holds the highest level of certification by the Yoga Alliance in the US and the UK (EYRT 500/Senior Teacher). She is a senior faculty member of triyoga's teacher-training programme and was key in creating the course and syllabus for the level 1 and restorative yoga teacher-training programmes. For information on her classes, workshops, retreats, meditation courses and her DVD *Yoga 3D – Interactive Learning with Anna Ashby* visit: www.annaashby.com

Lucy May Constantini

Lucy May Constantini has been practising yoga *asana* since 1992 and meditation since 1999. She taught for many years before undertaking her formal yoga teacher training at triyoga in London, which she passed with distinction in 2009. Lucy is a student of Kashmir Shaivism and Advaita Vedanta, as well as having undertaken meditation study in both the Tibetan and Theravada Buddhist traditions. She has studied in India and southeast Asia as well as the UK. lucymayconstantini.wordpress.com

Laura Denham Jones

Laura Denham Jones took up competitive distance running to keep fit in her 20s. Yoga added another dimension to her running – both physically and mentally – and it led to a change in career as a yoga teacher. She undertook teacher training at It's Yoga in San Francisco in 2001 and later with Shiva Rea in vinyasa flow. She has notched up eight marathons with a best time of 3.45, has pioneered triyoga's 'Yoga for Runners and Sports'

programme and teaches yoga for runners, cyclists and triathletes. www.yogaforrunners.co.uk

Ayala Gill

Ayala Gill began practising Iyengar yoga at age six and has been teaching for more than 15 years. She has a regular vipassana meditation practice and is inspired by Insight Yoga as a path of awakening. She draws from Buddhist, Tantric and modern psychotherapeutic wisdom to help her students integrate mind, body and spirit. Ayala's passion for pregnancy yoga began after the birth of the first of her three children in 1999. As a way of offering continuity for women between classes she has created the App 'Pregnancy Yoga with Ayala Gill', and extends this continuity to some students by acting as a doula (birth support) during their births. Ayala extends heartfelt gratitude to her teachers, who continually rekindle her commitment to living with intimacy and love.

Louise Grime

Louise Grime discovered yoga in 1978 as an antidote to the stress of her job managing restaurants. She spent time at the Sivananda Ashram in Kerala, where she completed her yoga teacher training and worked as a member of staff. She qualified as an Iyengar yoga teacher and studied at the Iyengar Yoga Institute in Pune, practised Shadow yoga with founder Zhander Remete and Ashtanga vinyasa with John Scott. She is author of the book and DVD *15-minute Gentle Yoga*, which has been translated into several languages. Louise teaches in London with regular classes at triyoga and The Life Centre. lakshmilou@hotmail.com

Jean Hall

Hearing tales of her mother's upbringing in Calcutta was the start of Jean Hall's curiosity for all things Indian. However, it wasn't until she trained as a dancer in her late teens that yoga began to feature in her life. She found that while dance often concentrates on

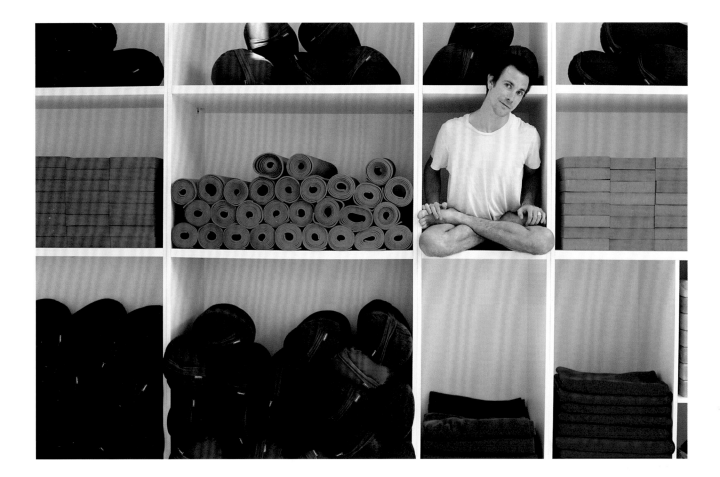

projecting energy and an image outwardly, yoga focuses on cultivating a deep internal sensory awareness of the body and mind. Her interest in yoga's 'subtle anatomy' and its network of energy pathways grew and now Jean teaches slow flow dynamic yoga to help students become mindful of these subtle aspects. She has written two books: *Yoga, a practical guide to yoga postures*, and *Astanga Yoga, an in-depth guide to the primary series* and is part of triyoga's teacher-training faculty. www.yogajeannie.com

Susannah Hoffman

Susannah Hoffman grew up surrounded by the philosophy of yoga. Her father had been initiated into Transcendental Meditation by the Maharishi Mahesh Yogi in 1961 and she remembers doing her first yoga postures at age four and 'wanting to be blue like Krishna'. When Susannah was 17, her mother took her to her first spiritual exercise class (a type of meditation).

She now teaches yoga to children and adults as well as pregnancy yoga and baby massage. She is part of the triyoga teacher-training team and has put together its Yoga For Children teacher-training programme. Her teenage son Marlowe sometimes assists her in classes and she thanks him for being a constant source of inspiration. www.susannahhoffmanyoga.com

Jane Kersel

Jane Kersal is an international coach and therapist specialising in integrative health, wellbeing and relationship: with ourselves, each other and in the corporate world. She uses yoga, meditation, energetic education, hypnotherapy, psychology, natural nutrition and Voice Dialogue to create positive shifts in her clients. One of the most respected UK yoga teachers and opinion formers, she has featured in the *Wall Street Journal*, *The Sunday Times* etc. She regularly works with entire families, where she shares the

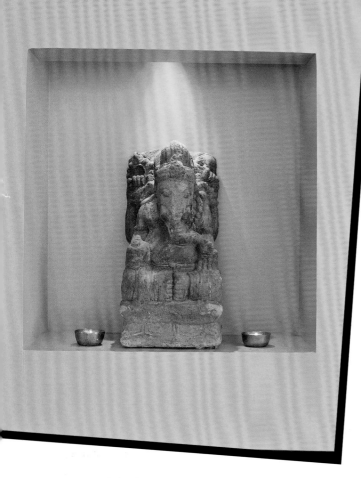

training course. Her classes interweave alignment-and-breath-based vinyasa flow, meditation, and yogic philosophy. She is also the author of the DVD *Vinyasa Yoga: A Steady, Mindful Practice*. www.mkdeemer.com

Timothy McCall

Timothy McCall MD is a board-certified specialist in internal medicine, the medical editor of *Yoga Journal* and the author of *Yoga as Medicine: The Yogic Prescription for Health and Healing*. He has studied yoga since 1995 with Patricia Walden, and more recently with Donald Moyer and Rod Stryker, as well as Ayurveda with a traditional Vaidyar (doctor) in Kerala, India. His teaching and writing focus on yoga therapy, holistic healing and on reconciling Eastern and Western ways of knowing. His teaching schedule and more than 100 archived articles, interviews, videos and podcasts can be found at www.DrMcCall.com

Joey Miles

Joey's big love (alongside his wife Donna and their two children, Caleb and Daisy) is Ashtanga yoga. He learnt this from his mentor Hamish Hendry in London and at the Sri K Pattabhi Jois Yoga Institute in Mysore, from the late Pattabhi Jois (Ashtanga's founder) himself. Latterly Joey has learnt from Jois' grandson Sharath. Joey lives in a small town in the Pennines and teaches both the Ashtanga led-class format as well as 'Mysore style'. He is part of triyoga's teacher-training faculty. www.ashtangayogaleeds.com

Nadia Narain

First embracing yoga to help restore balance to her fast-paced lifestyle, Nadia Narain is now one of the UK's most popular and best-loved yoga teachers. She draws on her study with some of the world's most renowned yoga and meditation teachers including Gurmukh Kaur Khalsa, with whom she trained in pregnancy yoga. She expanded her knowledge with Ina May Gaskin, author of *Spiritual Midwifery*, studying as an assistant midwife. She has attended numerous births and also acts as a doula (birth support). Nadia created triyoga's pregnancy teacher-training faculty and also teaches postnatal yoga. www.nadianarain.com

importance of consciousness work for building loving environments. She holds ERYT 500 certification (Yoga Alliance USA) and is acknowledged as a teacher's teacher with the British Wheel of Yoga. She also has certificates in pre- and postnatal yoga, hypnotherapy, natural nutrition and Voice Dialogue: The Psychology of the Selves and has sat on many yoga teaching faculties. www.janekersel.com

Mimi Kuo-Deemer

Mimi Kuo-Deemer began dabbling in yoga at a time when her main trajectory was documentary photography. A keen people watcher from an early age, she yearned to make better sense of people's behaviour and her place in the world. In time, she found that both photography and yoga were art forms that helped shed light into the complex nature of human interaction, relationships, and the Self. Mimi is the co-founder of Yoga Yard, a studio in Beijing. She is now based in London, and teaches on triyoga's teacher-

Alaric Newcombe

Alaric Newcombe has been practising Iyengar yoga since 1983 and is certificated as a Senior Intermediate level 3 Iyengar Yoga teacher, the highest qualification awarded by the Iyengar Yoga Association (UK), and as a teacher trainer. He has been taught by BKS Iyengar, and his son and daughter. Alaric's original teacher training was with the Mehta family. Alaric has a dynamic and flowing teaching style which is focused and insightful. His experience enables him to give precise individual adjustments and maintain group focus. He challenges inertia and ignorance with humour and compassion. He is also psychotherapist and group facilitator and maintains a small professional practice. www.alaricyoga.com

Jeff Phenix

Jeff Phenix has been practising yoga and meditation for more than 15 years and is a mentor and teacher on triyoga's teacher-training programme. He enjoys incorporating diverse themes, postures, sequences and yogic techniques creatively to help students improve their practice and deepen their understanding. He is influenced by a wide range of yoga styles – the emphasis on breath and movement of vinyasa flow, the precision of Iyengar yoga, the heart-orientated grace of Anusara, the individualised aspect of viniyoga and the traditional philosophy and spirituality of the Jivamukti and Satyananda schools. www.phenixyoga.com

Carlos Pomeda

Carlos Pomeda received formal, traditional training in yoga during almost 18 years as a monk of the Sarasvati order, nine of which he spent in India, in the Siddha Yoga Ashram, studying and practising under the guidance of Swami Muktananda and Gurumayi Chidvilasananda. During this time he learned the various systems of Indian philosophy, immersed himself in the practice of yoga and became one of the senior teaching monks of the tradition – teaching meditation and philosophy to tens of thousands of students around the world. He has a masters in Sanskrit from UC Berkeley and another in religious studies, from UC Santa Barbara. His set of six DVD's titled *The Wisdom*

of Yoga is a series of practical workshops on the history, philosophy and practices of the yoga tradition. Carlos is also part of triyoga's teacher-training faculty. www.pomeda.com

Amme Poulton

A former lawyer, Amme Poulton came to yoga seeking a low-impact exercise following surgery on both knees. After completing an ashtanga training in San Francisco in 2001, she began teaching yoga full-time. She completed a hatha training in 2003, and Ana Forrest's advanced training in 2000 and holds the highest Yoga Alliance UK certification. She taught in San Francisco for seven years before heading to London via Mexico and NYC. Her classes are challenging and dynamic, creating a practice that heals and detoxifies the body and mind. www.windinhair.com

John Stirk

Osteopath John Stirk was introduced to yoga in 1973 when he met his yoga teacher wife, Lolly. He was struck by the way it healed him on a physical and mental level in only a short space of time. In 1989, he began to study with Vanda Scaravelli. John is the author of several books on yoga and teaches internationally. His main interest is in Eastern and Western approaches to personal growth and his grounding in yoga, osteopathy and psychology has stimulated a continuously evolving style of teaching that gives space for insight and realisation to emerge. www.johnstirk.com

Bridget Woods-Kramer

Bridget Woods-Kramer came to yoga in the 1970s as a counterbalance to her highly successful but stressful career as the head of a fashion company and founder of leading wellbeing facilities (The Fitness Centre and ground-breaking day spa The Sanctuary in London). She embarked on an intense programme of study to become a senior teacher and teacher trainer. She has studied with Anusara's founder, John Friend, since 1994 and became a certified Anusara teacher in 2001. Bridget runs Anusara immersions and teacher trainings worldwide and the Anusara teacher-training programme for triyoga. www.bridgetwoodskramer.com

footnotes

History of Yoga
[1] *The Yoga Sutras* II.46
[2] Gita Desai, *Yoga Unveiled DVD*, 2004

The Eight Limbs of Yoga
[1] *The Yoga Sutras* II.52–53
[2] Ibid II.54–55

Yoga for Health
[1] Trisha Lamb, http://www.iayt.org/site_Vx2/publications/articles/hlthbenefits.aspx, 2004
[2] www.ornishspectrum.com
[3] www.sciatica.org/yoga/study_overview.html

Yoga for Men
[1] www.mindbodygreen.com/0-1995/Q-A-with-Baron-Baptiste-Kids-Men-Yoga-More.html
[2] Interview with Lucy Kellaway, *The Financial Times, FT Weekend Magazine*, 23rd April 2011
[3] www.yogajournal.com/lifestyle/2585
[4] http://www.telegraph.co.uk/health/wellbeing/8867059/Power-yoga-how-money-has-changed-a-spiritual-pursuit.html
[5] Interview with Jonathan Northcroft, *The Sunday Times*, 17th January 2010.
[6] Timothy McCall MD, *Yoga as Medicine*, Bantam, 2007, p.7
[7] *Yoga for Healing and Happiness*, Yoga Journal, 2011, p.8

Yoga for Women
[1] http://171.67.121.89/content/29/2/207.abstract
[2] *The Practice of Women During the Whole Month*, downloadable from iyengaryoga.org.uk
[3] Dr Claudia Welch, *Balance Your Hormones, Balance Your Life* (Da Capo Press) 2011, p.32
[4] Menopause Awareness Alliance Survey, cited in *Your Change Your Choice* (Hodder Mobius) 2006, Michael Dooley & Sarah Stacey, p.41,
[5] Studies by Robert Freedman, Wayne State University School of Medicine, cited in *Your Change Your Choice* (Hodder Mobius) 2006, Michael Dooley & Sarah Stacey, p.79

Yoga for Relationships
[1] Erich Schifmann, *Yoga: the Spirit and Practice of Moving into Stillness* (Pocket Books) 1996
[2] Donna Farhi, *Bringing Yoga to Life* (HarperOne) 2003, p.59
[3] *The Yoga-Sutra of Patanjali* (Shambhala Publications) 2003, translated by Chip Hartranft

Energy
[1] Hiroshi Motoyama, Ph.D., 'Acupuncture Meridians exist in Dermis (Connective Tissues) – Comparative studies of Electrical Potential Gradient and Direction of Current Flow in Epidermis and Dermis', *CIHS Journal* 2008, Vol 3 No.1
[2] BKS Iyengar, *Iyengar Yoga For Beginners* (Dorling Kindersley) 2006, p.33.

Meditation
[1] Full Catastrophe Living: How to cope with stress, pain and illness using mindfulness meditation by J Kabat-Zinn, Piatkus 1990 (pp69-70). As cited in the 'Mindfulness Report' 2010, by The Mental Health Foundation.
[2] Point 1.4.4.2. NICE recommends Mindfulness Based Cognitive Therapy for people with a history of depression at risk of relapse. 'Common mental health disorders: Identification and pathways to care', NICE clinical guideline 123, May 2011.
[3] Matthieu Ricard, *The Art of Meditation* (Atlantic Books) 2010, p.15
[4] 'The restraint of the modifications of the mind-stuff is Yoga/ Then the Seer abides in his own nature.' Book, sutras 2–3. The Yoga Sutras of Patanjali, translation and commentary by Sri Swami Satchidananda, Integral Yoga Publications 1990, pp.3–6.
[5] Sally Kempton, *Meditation for the Love of It* (Sounds True) 2010, p.36
[6] Ibid p.43
[7] Ibid p.26
[8] Ibid p.23
[9] Matthieu Ricard, *The Art of Meditation* (Atlantic Books) 2010, p.13
[10] Ibid p16.

contact details

triyoga centres in London:
Primrose Hill: 6 erskine road, primrose hill, nw3 3aj
Chelsea: 372 king's road, chelsea, sw3 5uz
Soho: 2nd floor, kingly court, soho, w1b 5pw
Covent Garden: wallacespace, 2 dryden street, covent garden, wc2e 9na

Tel: 020 7483 3344
www.triyoga.co.uk

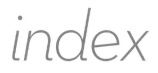

credits

Kyle Books would like to thank the following for providing photographs and permission to reproduce copyright material. While every effort has been made to trace and acknowledge all copyright holders, we would like to apologise should there have been any errors or omissions.

p.4, Yangshuo, iStock Photo
pp.8 (b.r.), 26 (t.r), 112, Victoria Woodhall
p.14, Indian School, Getty Images
pp.23, 40, 132–133, 142 (inset), 152 (inset), 156 (inset), John Penberthy

p.24 (m.l), Boston Globe, Getty Images; (b.r) Matt Cardy, Getty Images
p.27 (t.l.), Govinda Kai
p.28 (t.l.), Lucy Wallace
p.35 (m.b.), EyesWideOpen, Getty Images
p.60 (b.l.), yogacity.nl
p.72 (author pic), Karen Yeomans
p.80 (b.l.), Masakazu Watanabe/Aflo, Getty Images; (b.m.), photomorphic, iStock Photo; (b.r.), Bert Design, Getty Images
p.86 (b.l.), Rob Howard
p.87 (spine), Hulton Archive, Getty Images
p.100 (author pic), Michal Venera
p.129, Aaron Deemer
p.172 (chakras), Veena Mari, iStock Photo

Key: t = top, m = middle, b = bottom, l = left, r = right

index

acknowledgements

Victoria:

To my friends and colleagues for putting up with my 'yoga bore' moments. To my editor at *YOU*, Sue Peart, for allowing me to take on this project in the first place, and to everyone who supports my Tuesday classes at Northcliffe House – you have helped me to develop knowledge and practice. To Jonathan for trusting me with his brand, tolerating my crack-of-dawn meetings and being fun to work with (not forgetting golden retriever JayJay for keeping him on the leash). To the triyoga teachers for giving me so much of their precious time and inspiring expertise. To Kyle, all her team and my editor Catharine for keeping the many strands of this ambitious project on track and daring to suggest a DVD (for which thank you to our 'models' Mirja, Nina, Jennifer, Vance, Giti, Chris, Susanne and Jaqueline, and to Primrose Hill Centre Manager, Lauren, for smiling through all the disruption). The super-talented Angela Lamb for her brilliant layouts and long-standing Sagittarian friendship and Clare Park for her photography which makes yoga look like fun, not homework. Thank you Liz Murray for copy editing and Sarah Stacey (author, with Michael Dooley, of *Your Change Your Choice*) for help with the menopause section. To Michelle, Nina and my Tuesday class for testing out the sequences and making pertinent suggestions. To Amir Jaan for advice on Kundalini yoga, Tim Cummins for help with Shadow yoga and Sissi Gill for her expertise in never-too-late yoga and her elegant poses in the 'yoga for women' section alongside daughter Ayala and granddaughter Elsa. Namaste to Lara Baumann at Quantum Yoga for inspiring me to take teacher training. Thank you to Asquith for providing the most comfortable and stylish yoga clothes (as modelled by Bridget and me). To Dorothee, Sarah and Ana – your bumps really made the pregnancy section. To the superstar yogi children: Marlowe, Julien, Lyla, Rose, Heather, Delilah, Jasper, Amber, Anja and Alexandra and to my own two angels, Marcus and Clara, who let me take what should have been family time to write this book. Kids – I hope you'll realise how special you are to me when you look at these pages in years to come. To my mum Viola, for lifelong love, concern and support, my father Michael for proofreading, NLP and for taking up Bournemouth beach yoga as moral support. And most of all to Matthew – husband and yoga refusenik – for stepping up with childcare, cooking and general cheerleading to allow me to pursue my dream project.

Jonathan:

Many dittos to the above and, of course, Victoria for sharing the vision and making it happen. To all triyoga in-house and guest teachers and staff past, present and future who have contributed so much to the triyoga experience; to Lee and Bridget and Teddy and Scout for being the catalysts; to Clare Park for such great photography; to Jane for so much; to the triyoga investors who believed in what we wanted to create: Simon, Georgie, Tina and Ford; to Emma and Matt at 23 for keeping us in line where they could; to JayJay and triyoga therapists for keeping the office (Rachel, Paul, Jennifer, Nina, Marinos et al.) sane/healthy most of the time; to John Stirk for being my first real *asana* teacher and above all to my teacher Gurumayi for giving me so much.

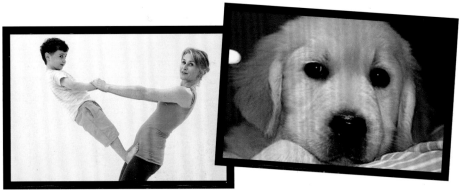

Victoria and her son Marcus

Jonathan's dog, JayJay